Chapter 1: Understanding Pituitary Tumors

What are Pituitary Tumors?

Pituitary tumors are abnormal growths that develop in the pituitary gland, a small pea-sized gland located at the base of the brain. These tumors can be either benign (noncancerous) or malignant (cancerous) and can cause a variety of symptoms depending on their size and location. Understanding pituitary tumors is crucial for patients who are navigating a diagnosis and exploring treatment options.

Treatment options for pituitary tumors vary depending on the type of tumor, its size, and the symptoms it is causing. Some common treatment approaches include surgery, radiation therapy, and medication. Each patient's treatment plan will be tailored to their individual needs and may involve a combination of these modalities.

Managing symptoms of pituitary tumors is an important aspect of treatment and can help improve quality of life for patients. Symptoms may include headaches, vision changes, hormone imbalances, and fatigue. Working closely with a healthcare team to address these symptoms and manage any hormonal imbalances is essential for optimal outcomes.

Surgical interventions for pituitary tumors may be recommended to remove the tumor and alleviate pressure on the surrounding structures in the brain. Minimally invasive surgical techniques are often used to minimize the risk of complications and reduce recovery time. Patients should discuss the risks and benefits of surgery with their healthcare provider to make an informed decision.

Non-invasive treatment methods, such as medication and radiation therapy, may be used for patients who are not candidates for surgery or who prefer a less invasive approach. These treatments can help shrink the tumor, alleviate symptoms, and prevent recurrence. It is important for patients to discuss all available treatment options with their healthcare team to determine the best course of action for their individual situation.

Types of Pituitary Tumors

There are several types of pituitary tumors that can affect individuals, each with its own set of characteristics and treatment options. The most common type of pituitary tumor is known as a pituitary adenoma, which is a noncancerous growth that develops in the pituitary gland. Pituitary adenomas can be classified based on their size and hormone-secreting abilities, leading to various symptoms and treatment approaches.

Another type of pituitary tumor is called a craniopharyngioma, which originates from embryonic tissue near the pituitary gland. These tumors can be large and cause pressure on surrounding structures, leading to symptoms such as headaches, vision changes, and hormonal imbalances. Treatment for craniopharyngiomas often involves a combination of surgery, radiation therapy, and hormone replacement therapy.

Rarer types of pituitary tumors include Rathke's cleft cysts, chordomas, and metastatic tumors that have spread to the pituitary gland from other parts of the body. These tumors may require specialized treatment approaches and close monitoring to manage symptoms and prevent complications. It is essential for patients to work closely with a multidisciplinary team of healthcare providers to determine the most appropriate treatment plan for their specific type of pituitary tumor.

In some cases, pituitary tumors may be classified as functioning or nonfunctioning based on their hormone-secreting abilities. Functioning tumors produce excess hormones that can lead to a variety of symptoms, while nonfunctioning tumors do not produce hormones but can still cause symptoms due to their size and location.

Understanding the type of pituitary tumor you have is crucial in determining the most effective treatment approach and managing potential complications.

Overall, having a clear understanding of the different types of pituitary tumors can help patients navigate their diagnosis and treatment options more effectively. By working closely with a team of healthcare providers and staying informed about the characteristics of their specific tumor, patients can make informed decisions about their care and improve their quality of life. It is important for patients to seek out support resources and stay proactive in managing their condition to achieve the best possible outcomes.

Causes and Risk Factors

Pituitary tumors are abnormal growths that develop in the pituitary gland, a small pea-sized gland located at the base of the brain. These tumors can be either noncancerous (benign) or cancerous (malignant) and can cause a variety of symptoms depending on their size and location. Understanding the causes and risk factors associated with pituitary tumors is essential for patients navigating their diagnosis and treatment.

The exact cause of pituitary tumors is not always clear, but certain risk factors have been identified that may increase the likelihood of developing these growths. One common risk factor is a family history of pituitary tumors or other genetic conditions that predispose individuals to developing tumors in the pituitary gland. Additionally, hormonal imbalances, such as excess production of certain hormones like prolactin or growth hormone, can also contribute to the development of pituitary tumors.

Genetic factors play a significant role in the development of pituitary tumors, with certain genetic mutations increasing the risk of tumor formation in the pituitary gland. Patients with a family history of pituitary tumors or genetic syndromes such as multiple endocrine neoplasia type 1 (MEN1) or Carney complex may be at a higher risk of developing these growths. It is important for patients with a family history of pituitary tumors to undergo regular screening and monitoring to detect any potential tumors early.

In addition to genetic factors, certain hormonal imbalances can also contribute to the development of pituitary tumors. For example, overproduction of growth hormone (acromegaly) or prolactin (prolactinoma) can lead to the formation of tumors in the pituitary gland. These hormonal imbalances can be caused by a variety of factors, including pituitary adenomas, which are the most common type of pituitary tumors.

Overall, understanding the causes and risk factors associated with pituitary tumors is crucial for patients navigating their diagnosis and treatment. By identifying these factors early on, healthcare providers can develop personalized treatment plans that address the underlying causes of the tumors and help patients manage their symptoms effectively. Patients with a family history of pituitary tumors or genetic syndromes should work closely with their healthcare team to monitor their condition and explore treatment options that best suit their needs.

Common Symptoms

One of the most common symptoms of pituitary tumors is headaches. These headaches are often persistent and may be severe in nature. Patients may experience dull, aching pain that is localized to the front of the head or behind the eyes. In some cases, these headaches may be accompanied by visual disturbances such as blurry vision or double vision. It is important to note that not all headaches are indicative of a pituitary tumor, but if you are experiencing frequent or severe headaches, it is important to consult with a healthcare provider.

Another common symptom of pituitary tumors is changes in vision. This can manifest as blurry or double vision, tunnel vision, or even loss of peripheral vision. These changes in vision are typically caused by the tumor pressing on the optic nerves or optic chiasm, which can lead to visual disturbances. It is important to seek medical attention if you are experiencing any changes in your vision, as early detection and treatment of pituitary tumors can help prevent further complications.

Hormonal imbalances are also common symptoms of pituitary tumors. Depending on the type of tumor and its location, patients may experience a variety of hormonal changes. For example, tumors that produce excess hormones may cause symptoms such as weight gain, fatigue, muscle weakness, and mood swings. On the other hand, tumors that disrupt hormone production may lead to symptoms such as infertility, irregular menstrual cycles, and decreased libido. It is important for patients to undergo hormone testing to identify any imbalances and develop a targeted treatment plan.

In addition to headaches, vision changes, and hormonal imbalances, pituitary tumors can also cause symptoms such as nausea, vomiting, and fatigue. These symptoms may be nonspecific and can often be attributed to other conditions, which can make diagnosis challenging. Patients with pituitary tumors may also experience symptoms related to the compression of nearby structures, such as sinus congestion, difficulty swallowing, or changes in facial appearance. It is important for patients to communicate any new or worsening symptoms to their healthcare provider to ensure timely diagnosis and appropriate treatment.

Overall, it is important for patients to be aware of the common symptoms associated with pituitary tumors and to seek medical attention if they are experiencing any of these symptoms. Early detection and treatment of pituitary tumors can help improve outcomes and quality of life for patients. By working closely with a healthcare provider and being proactive about monitoring symptoms, patients can navigate the diagnosis and treatment of pituitary tumors with confidence and support.

Diagnosis and Screening

Diagnosis and screening are crucial steps in the management of pituitary tumors. Early detection can lead to more effective treatment options and better outcomes for patients. When it comes to navigating pituitary tumors, understanding the diagnostic process is key.

In order to diagnose a pituitary tumor, your healthcare provider may recommend a variety of tests and screenings. These can include blood tests to check hormone levels, imaging studies such as MRI or CT scans to visualize the tumor, and vision tests to assess any impact on the optic nerve. It is important to work closely with your healthcare team to determine the best course of action based on your individual case.

Once a pituitary tumor has been diagnosed, treatment options will be discussed. These can range from surgical interventions to non-invasive treatment methods, depending on the size and location of the tumor. Managing symptoms of pituitary tumors is also an important aspect of treatment, as hormonal imbalances caused by the tumor can lead to a variety of physical and emotional challenges.

Surgical interventions for pituitary tumors may be necessary to remove the tumor and alleviate pressure on surrounding structures. Your healthcare provider will discuss the risks and benefits of surgery, as well as any potential long-term effects. Non-invasive treatment methods, such as medication or radiation therapy, may also be considered as part of a comprehensive treatment plan.

Throughout the diagnosis and treatment process, it is important to consider the impact of pituitary tumors on mental health and well-being. Support resources for patients with pituitary tumors can provide valuable assistance and guidance. Additionally, understanding genetic factors related to pituitary tumors and potential strategies for prevention can help patients take control of their health and future.

Chapter 2: Navigating Pituitary Tumors

Finding the Right Healthcare Team

Finding the right healthcare team is crucial when it comes to navigating the complexities of pituitary tumors. Your healthcare team will play a vital role in guiding you through the diagnosis and treatment process, as well as helping you manage the symptoms and side effects associated with this condition. It is important to find healthcare professionals who are experienced in treating pituitary tumors and who can provide you with the support and care you need.

When looking for the right healthcare team, it is important to consider the different treatment options available for pituitary tumors. Your healthcare team should be knowledgeable about the various surgical interventions, non-invasive treatment methods, and hormonal therapies that may be recommended for your specific type of tumor. They should also be able to discuss the potential long-term effects of treatment and help you make informed decisions about your care.

Managing symptoms of pituitary tumors can be challenging, but having a supportive healthcare team by your side can make a big difference. Your healthcare providers should work with you to develop a personalized treatment plan that addresses your symptoms and improves your quality of life. They should also be able to help you navigate any hormonal imbalances that may arise as a result of your tumor.

In addition to providing medical care, your healthcare team should also be able to offer support resources to help you cope with the emotional and psychological impact of pituitary tumors. They should be able to connect you with support groups, mental health professionals, and other resources that can help you maintain your mental health and well-being throughout your treatment journey.

By finding the right healthcare team, you can feel confident that you are receiving the best possible care for your pituitary tumor. Your healthcare providers should be dedicated to helping you achieve the best possible outcomes and should work with you to develop a comprehensive treatment plan that meets your individual needs. Remember, you are not alone in this journey – your healthcare team is here to support you every step of the way.

Treatment Centers and Facilities

Treatment centers and facilities play a crucial role in the management of pituitary tumors. These centers are equipped with specialized medical professionals who have expertise in diagnosing and treating pituitary tumors. Patients can benefit from the comprehensive care provided at these facilities, which often include a multidisciplinary approach involving endocrinologists, neurosurgeons, radiation oncologists, and other healthcare providers.

When it comes to navigating pituitary tumors, patients have a range of treatment options available to them. These may include surgical interventions, non-invasive treatments such as medication or radiation therapy, and hormonal therapy to address imbalances caused by the tumor. The choice of treatment will depend on the type and size of the tumor, as well as the patient's overall health and preferences.

Managing symptoms of pituitary tumors is an important aspect of treatment, and treatment centers often provide supportive care to help patients cope with the physical and emotional challenges of living with a pituitary tumor. This may include managing side effects of treatment, addressing hormonal imbalances, and providing resources for emotional support and mental health care.

Surgical interventions are often necessary for the treatment of pituitary tumors, and treatment centers may offer minimally invasive approaches such as endoscopic surgery to remove the tumor. These procedures are aimed at preserving normal pituitary function while effectively removing the tumor and alleviating symptoms. Patients can expect thorough pre-operative evaluation and post-operative care to ensure the best possible outcome.

In addition to surgical interventions, treatment centers may also offer non-invasive treatment methods such as radiation therapy or medication to manage pituitary tumors. These treatments are designed to target the tumor while minimizing damage to surrounding tissues. Patients can work closely with their healthcare team to develop a personalized treatment plan that takes into account their specific needs and goals.

Insurance Coverage and Financial Considerations

Insurance coverage and financial considerations are important aspects to consider when navigating the diagnosis and treatment of pituitary tumors. As a patient, it is crucial to understand what your insurance plan covers in terms of diagnostic tests, medical consultations, surgeries, medications, and follow-up care related to pituitary tumors. It is essential to review your insurance policy and communicate with your healthcare provider to ensure that you are aware of any potential out-of-pocket costs and financial responsibilities.

Treatment options for pituitary tumors can vary depending on the size, location, and type of tumor. Some common treatment approaches include surgery, radiation therapy, and medication. It is important to discuss the potential costs associated with each treatment option with your healthcare provider and insurance company. Understanding your insurance coverage for these treatments can help you make informed decisions about your care while also managing your financial obligations.

Managing symptoms of pituitary tumors may require ongoing medical care, including regular doctor visits, imaging tests, and hormone replacement therapy. It is important to discuss with your healthcare provider how your insurance coverage can help offset the costs of managing these symptoms. Additionally, some insurance plans may offer coverage for alternative therapies such as acupuncture or physical therapy, which can also help alleviate symptoms associated with pituitary tumors.

Surgical interventions for pituitary tumors are often necessary to remove the tumor and alleviate symptoms. It is essential to understand the potential costs associated with surgery, including hospital fees, surgeon fees, anesthesia, and post-operative care. Your insurance coverage may help cover some or all of these costs, but it is important to verify coverage with your insurance provider before undergoing surgery.

In conclusion, understanding your insurance coverage and financial considerations is an important part of navigating the diagnosis and treatment of pituitary tumors. By being proactive in reviewing your insurance policy, communicating with your healthcare provider, and exploring all available treatment options, you can make informed decisions about your care while also managing the financial impact of treatment. Remember to advocate for yourself and seek out resources and support to help you through this journey.

Second Opinions and Advocacy

When facing a diagnosis of a pituitary tumor, it is essential for patients to seek second opinions from qualified medical professionals. While your primary care physician or initial specialist may have provided valuable insight into your condition, obtaining a second opinion can offer a fresh perspective and potentially uncover additional treatment options. Seeking a second opinion does not signify a lack of trust in your current healthcare provider, but rather demonstrates a proactive approach to understanding and managing your condition.

Advocacy plays a crucial role in navigating the complex landscape of pituitary tumors. As a patient, it is important to advocate for yourself and ensure that your voice is heard throughout the diagnostic and treatment process. This may involve asking questions, seeking clarification on medical recommendations, and actively participating in decision-making regarding your care. By advocating for yourself, you can play an active role in shaping your treatment plan and ensuring that your unique needs and preferences are taken into account.

In some cases, patients may encounter conflicting opinions or treatment recommendations from different healthcare providers. In such instances, it is important to carefully weigh the information provided by each professional and consider seeking a third opinion if necessary. Consulting with multiple experts can help you make informed decisions about your care and choose the treatment approach that aligns best with your goals and values.

In addition to seeking multiple opinions, patients may also benefit from engaging with advocacy organizations and support groups focused on pituitary tumors. These resources can provide valuable information, emotional support, and practical guidance for navigating the challenges associated with the condition. By connecting with others who have firsthand experience with pituitary tumors, patients can gain insights into coping strategies, treatment options, and ways to enhance their overall well-being.

Ultimately, by proactively seeking second opinions, advocating for themselves, and engaging with supportive resources, patients can empower themselves to take an active role in managing their pituitary tumor diagnosis. By approaching their care with a sense of agency and resilience, patients can navigate the complexities of treatment options, symptom management, and long-term effects with confidence and clarity.

Clinical Trials and Research Opportunities

Clinical trials and research opportunities are essential components of advancing the understanding and treatment of pituitary tumors. Patients diagnosed with pituitary tumors may have the opportunity to participate in clinical trials that can offer innovative treatment options and contribute to the development of new therapies. These trials often involve testing the effectiveness and safety of new medications, surgical techniques, or non-invasive treatment methods.

Navigating the world of clinical trials can be overwhelming for patients, but it is important to remember that participation in these studies can potentially benefit not only the individual patient but also future patients facing similar diagnoses. By participating in a clinical trial, patients can play an active role in shaping the future of pituitary tumor treatment and contribute to the advancement of medical knowledge in this field.

Research opportunities related to pituitary tumors are constantly evolving, with new studies and trials being conducted to explore different aspects of diagnosis, treatment, and management of these tumors. Patients interested in participating in research studies should consult with their healthcare providers to learn about available opportunities and determine if they are eligible to participate.

It is important for patients to carefully consider the risks and benefits of participating in a clinical trial or research study. Healthcare providers can help patients understand the potential outcomes of participating in a trial and provide guidance on making informed decisions about whether to participate. Patients should also discuss any concerns or questions they may have with their healthcare team before committing to participate in a trial.

Overall, clinical trials and research opportunities offer patients with pituitary tumors the chance to access cutting-edge treatment options, contribute to the advancement of medical knowledge, and potentially improve outcomes for themselves and future patients. By staying informed about available opportunities and working closely with their healthcare providers, patients can make informed decisions about participating in clinical trials and research studies that align with their treatment goals and preferences.

Chapter 3: Treatment Options for Pituitary Tumors

Surgery

Surgery is a common treatment option for patients with pituitary tumors, particularly those that are large or causing significant symptoms. The goal of surgery is to remove as much of the tumor as possible while preserving normal pituitary function and minimizing the risk of complications. There are several surgical approaches that may be used depending on the size and location of the tumor, including transsphenoidal surgery, craniotomy, and endoscopic surgery.

Transsphenoidal surgery is the most common approach for removing pituitary tumors. During this procedure, the surgeon accesses the pituitary gland through the nasal cavity and removes the tumor using specialized instruments. This minimally invasive approach typically results in shorter hospital stays, faster recovery times, and fewer complications compared to traditional open surgery techniques.

In some cases, a craniotomy may be necessary to remove larger or more complex pituitary tumors. This involves making an incision in the skull to access the tumor directly. While craniotomies are more invasive and carry a higher risk of complications, they may be the best option for certain patients with tumors that are difficult to reach using other surgical approaches.

Endoscopic surgery is a newer technique that allows surgeons to remove pituitary tumors through the nose using a small camera and specialized instruments. This approach offers improved visualization of the tumor and surrounding structures, leading to more precise tumor removal and lower rates of complications. Endoscopic surgery is becoming increasingly popular for the treatment of pituitary tumors due to its effectiveness and minimal invasiveness.

Overall, surgery can be an effective treatment option for patients with pituitary tumors, particularly when other treatments have not been successful or are not appropriate. It is important for patients to discuss the risks and benefits of surgery with their healthcare team and to carefully consider their options before proceeding. With advances in surgical techniques and technology, many patients are able to undergo successful tumor removal with minimal side effects and improved quality of life.

Radiation Therapy

Radiation therapy is a common treatment option for patients with pituitary tumors, particularly those who have residual or recurrent tumors after surgery. This form of therapy uses high-energy radiation to target and destroy tumor cells, either by shrinking the tumor or stopping its growth. Radiation therapy can be delivered externally, through a machine that directs radiation beams at the tumor from outside the body, or internally, using radioactive materials placed directly into or near the tumor.

External beam radiation therapy is often used for pituitary tumors that cannot be completely removed through surgery, or for tumors that are located close to critical structures in the brain. This type of radiation therapy is usually given in daily doses over a period of several weeks, with the goal of delivering a precise amount of radiation to the tumor while minimizing damage to surrounding healthy tissue. Internal radiation therapy, also known as brachytherapy, involves placing radioactive seeds or pellets directly into the tumor or nearby tissue. This allows for a more targeted dose of radiation to be delivered to the tumor, while reducing the risk of damage to surrounding structures.

One of the benefits of radiation therapy for pituitary tumors is its ability to control tumor growth and reduce symptoms, even in cases where surgery is not an option. Radiation therapy can also be used as adjuvant therapy after surgery, to target any remaining tumor cells and reduce the risk of recurrence. However, like any form of treatment, radiation therapy carries potential risks and side effects, including fatigue, hair loss, skin irritation, and damage to nearby structures in the brain. It is important for patients to discuss these risks and benefits with their healthcare team before deciding on a treatment plan.

In addition to its role in treating pituitary tumors, radiation therapy can also be used to manage symptoms caused by hormonal imbalances. For example, radiation therapy can be targeted at specific areas of the pituitary gland to reduce hormone production and alleviate symptoms such as excessive thirst, urination, or fatigue. This approach may be particularly beneficial for patients with pituitary tumors that are resistant to other forms of treatment, or for those who are not candidates for surgery. As with any treatment option, it is important for patients to weigh the potential benefits and risks of radiation therapy in the context of their overall health and treatment goals.

Overall, radiation therapy is an important tool in the management of pituitary tumors, offering patients a non-invasive treatment option that can effectively target tumor cells and reduce symptoms. By working closely with their healthcare team to develop a personalized treatment plan, patients can navigate the complexities of pituitary tumor treatment and make informed decisions about their care. With ongoing monitoring and support, patients can effectively manage their condition and improve their quality of life in the long term.

Medication

Medication plays a crucial role in the management of pituitary tumors, as it can help control symptoms, reduce tumor size, and regulate hormone levels. Patients with pituitary tumors may be prescribed a variety of medications, depending on the type of tumor they have and the symptoms they are experiencing. It is important for patients to work closely with their healthcare team to understand the purpose of each medication, how to take it properly, and any potential side effects to watch out for.

One common type of medication used to treat pituitary tumors is dopamine agonists, which can help shrink certain types of tumors and reduce the production of prolactin. These medications are typically taken orally and may need to be adjusted over time based on the patient's response to treatment. Another type of medication commonly used for pituitary tumors is somatostatin analogs, which can help reduce hormone production and slow tumor growth. Patients may also be prescribed hormone replacement therapy to address any hormonal imbalances caused by the tumor or its treatment.

In addition to medications specifically targeted at treating the tumor itself, patients with pituitary tumors may also need medications to manage symptoms such as headaches, vision changes, and hormonal imbalances. These medications can help improve quality of life and alleviate discomfort while undergoing treatment for the tumor. It is important for patients to communicate openly with their healthcare team about any symptoms they are experiencing so that appropriate medications can be prescribed.

It is important for patients to take their medications as prescribed and to follow up regularly with their healthcare team to monitor their progress. Some medications may need to be adjusted over time based on the patient's response and any changes in their condition. Patients should also be aware of potential side effects of their medications and report any concerns to their healthcare provider promptly.

Overall, medication is an important component of treatment for pituitary tumors and can play a significant role in helping patients manage their condition and improve their quality of life. By working closely with their healthcare team and following their treatment plan, patients can optimize the effectiveness of their medications and achieve the best possible outcomes in their journey to navigate and treat their pituitary tumor.

Watchful Waiting

Watchful waiting is a common approach in the management of pituitary tumors, especially for those with non-functioning tumors that are not causing any symptoms or pressing on surrounding structures. This strategy involves closely monitoring the tumor with regular imaging tests to track its size and growth rate over time. By opting for watchful waiting, patients can avoid unnecessary treatment interventions and potential side effects until the tumor shows signs of progression.

During the watchful waiting period, it is important for patients to maintain open communication with their healthcare team and adhere to scheduled follow-up appointments. These visits may include physical exams, blood tests to monitor hormone levels, and imaging studies such as MRI or CT scans. By staying informed and actively participating in their care, patients can better understand the status of their tumor and make informed decisions about potential treatment options if needed in the future.

While watchful waiting may be a suitable approach for some patients, it is crucial to be aware of any signs or symptoms that could indicate a change in the tumor's behavior. These may include headaches, vision changes, hormonal imbalances, or other neurological symptoms. If any new or worsening symptoms arise during the watchful waiting period, it is essential to promptly report them to your healthcare provider for further evaluation and potential treatment adjustments.

Patients undergoing watchful waiting for pituitary tumors should also focus on maintaining a healthy lifestyle to support overall well-being. This includes eating a balanced diet, engaging in regular physical activity, managing stress levels, and getting an adequate amount of sleep. By taking care of their physical and emotional health, patients can better cope with the uncertainties of watchful waiting and feel empowered in their journey towards managing their pituitary tumor.

In conclusion, watchful waiting is a valuable strategy for patients with pituitary tumors that do not require immediate intervention. By actively monitoring the tumor and staying connected with their healthcare team, patients can navigate the complexities of their diagnosis with confidence and clarity. Through education, communication, and self-care practices, patients can effectively manage their condition and make informed decisions about their treatment journey.

Combination Therapies

Combination therapies are often used in the treatment of pituitary tumors to maximize effectiveness and improve outcomes. These therapies involve the use of multiple treatment modalities in conjunction with one another to target the tumor from different angles. By combining different approaches, healthcare providers can better control the tumor growth and manage symptoms more effectively.

One common combination therapy for pituitary tumors is the use of surgery followed by radiation therapy. Surgical interventions are often used to remove as much of the tumor as possible, while radiation therapy is used to target any remaining tumor cells that may be left behind. This combination approach can help to reduce the risk of tumor recurrence and improve long-term outcomes for patients.

Another combination therapy that is often used for pituitary tumors is the use of surgery followed by hormonal therapy. Hormonal imbalances caused by pituitary tumors can have a significant impact on a patient's overall health and well-being. By using hormonal therapy in conjunction with surgery, healthcare providers can help to restore hormonal balance and improve symptoms such as fatigue, weight gain, and mood changes.

In some cases, combination therapies may also involve the use of non-invasive treatment methods such as stereotactic radiosurgery or drug therapy. These approaches can be used in combination with other treatment modalities to further enhance the effectiveness of the overall treatment plan. By tailoring the treatment approach to each individual patient's needs, healthcare providers can optimize outcomes and improve quality of life.

Overall, combination therapies offer a comprehensive and individualized approach to treating pituitary tumors. By combining different treatment modalities, healthcare providers can address the tumor from multiple angles and improve overall outcomes for patients. It is important for patients to work closely with their healthcare team to develop a treatment plan that is tailored to their specific needs and goals.

Chapter 4: Managing Symptoms of Pituitary Tumors

Headaches and Vision Changes

Headaches and vision changes are common symptoms experienced by patients with pituitary tumors. These symptoms can be caused by the tumor putting pressure on surrounding structures in the brain, such as the optic nerves. Patients may notice changes in their vision, including blurriness, double vision, or even loss of vision in severe cases. Headaches associated with pituitary tumors are often persistent and may be accompanied by nausea or vomiting.

It is important for patients to be aware of these symptoms and seek medical attention if they occur. Vision changes should be evaluated by an eye care specialist, while headaches should be discussed with a healthcare provider who is familiar with pituitary tumors. Early detection and treatment of these symptoms can help prevent further complications and improve the overall outcome for patients.

Treatment options for pituitary tumors may vary depending on the size and location of the tumor, as well as the patient's overall health and preferences. Surgical interventions, such as transsphenoidal surgery, may be recommended to remove the tumor and relieve pressure on surrounding structures. Non-invasive treatment methods, such as radiation therapy or medication, may also be considered to shrink the tumor and control hormone levels.

In some cases, pituitary tumors can cause hormonal imbalances that lead to a variety of symptoms, including fatigue, weight gain, and mood changes. These imbalances can be managed with hormone replacement therapy or other medications to help regulate hormone levels. Genetic factors may also play a role in the development of pituitary tumors, so it is important for patients to discuss their family history with their healthcare providers.

Managing symptoms of pituitary tumors can be challenging, but there are resources available to help patients navigate their diagnosis and treatment. Support groups, online forums, and patient advocacy organizations can provide valuable information and emotional support to patients and their families. It is important for patients to stay informed, ask questions, and advocate for their own healthcare needs throughout their journey with pituitary tumors.

Hormonal Imbalances

Hormonal imbalances are a common issue that can arise as a result of pituitary tumors. These tumors can disrupt the normal functioning of the pituitary gland, which plays a crucial role in regulating hormone production in the body. As a patient with a pituitary tumor, it is important to be aware of the potential hormonal imbalances that may occur and how they can impact your overall health.

One of the most common hormonal imbalances associated with pituitary tumors is hypersecretion of certain hormones, such as growth hormone or prolactin. This can lead to a range of symptoms, including abnormal growth, infertility, and changes in menstrual cycles. On the other hand, some pituitary tumors may result in hyposecretion of hormones, leading to issues such as fatigue, weight gain, and decreased libido. It is important to work closely with your healthcare team to monitor and manage these hormonal imbalances effectively.

In some cases, hormonal imbalances caused by pituitary tumors may require treatment through medication or hormone replacement therapy. Your healthcare provider will work with you to develop a personalized treatment plan that addresses your specific hormonal needs. It is crucial to follow your treatment plan diligently and communicate any changes in symptoms to your healthcare team.

Surgical interventions may also be necessary to address hormonal imbalances caused by pituitary tumors. Surgery can help to remove the tumor and restore normal hormone production in the pituitary gland. Your healthcare provider will discuss the potential risks and benefits of surgery with you and help you make an informed decision about your treatment options.

Overall, it is important for patients with pituitary tumors to be proactive in managing hormonal imbalances and seeking appropriate treatment. By working closely with your healthcare team, staying informed about your condition, and following your treatment plan, you can effectively manage hormonal imbalances and improve your overall health and well-being. Remember that you are not alone in this journey, and there are resources available to support you every step of the way.

Fatigue and Weakness

Fatigue and weakness are common symptoms experienced by patients with pituitary tumors. These symptoms can be caused by a variety of factors, including hormonal imbalances, the tumor's impact on normal bodily functions, and the stress of managing a chronic illness. It is important for patients to understand the underlying causes of their fatigue and weakness in order to effectively manage these symptoms.

One of the primary causes of fatigue and weakness in patients with pituitary tumors is hormonal imbalances. The pituitary gland plays a crucial role in regulating the body's hormones, and when a tumor develops in this gland, it can disrupt the normal production and release of hormones. This can lead to a range of symptoms, including fatigue, weakness, and low energy levels. Patients may also experience symptoms such as weight gain, muscle weakness, and mood changes as a result of hormonal imbalances caused by the tumor.

In addition to hormonal imbalances, the physical presence of a pituitary tumor can also contribute to fatigue and weakness. Tumors in the pituitary gland can put pressure on surrounding structures in the brain, leading to headaches, vision problems, and fatigue. The body may also divert energy and resources to fighting the tumor, leaving patients feeling tired and weak. It is important for patients to work closely with their healthcare team to address these physical symptoms and develop a comprehensive treatment plan.

Managing fatigue and weakness in patients with pituitary tumors often involves a combination of treatment options. This may include surgical interventions to remove the tumor, non-invasive treatment methods such as medication or radiation therapy, and lifestyle changes to improve overall health and well-being. Patients may also benefit from support resources, such as counseling or support groups, to help them cope with the emotional and mental impact of living with a pituitary tumor.

It is important for patients to be proactive in managing their symptoms of fatigue and weakness. This may involve keeping a symptom diary to track patterns and triggers, prioritizing rest and self-care, and communicating openly with their healthcare team about any changes or concerns. By taking an active role in their treatment and care, patients can better navigate the challenges of living with a pituitary tumor and improve their overall quality of life.

Cognitive Changes

Cognitive changes are a common symptom experienced by patients with pituitary tumors. These changes can manifest in various ways, including difficulty concentrating, memory problems, and changes in mood. It is important for patients to be aware of these cognitive changes and to seek appropriate medical guidance to address them.

One of the primary reasons for cognitive changes in patients with pituitary tumors is the impact of hormonal imbalances on the brain. The pituitary gland is responsible for producing and regulating hormones that are essential for proper brain function. When a tumor disrupts the normal function of the pituitary gland, it can lead to changes in hormone levels that affect cognitive abilities.

In addition to hormonal imbalances, cognitive changes may also be influenced by the location and size of the pituitary tumor. Tumors that grow larger or press against surrounding brain structures can interfere with cognitive processes, leading to symptoms such as confusion, slowed thinking, and difficulty processing information.

Managing cognitive changes associated with pituitary tumors often involves a combination of treatment options, including surgical interventions, non-invasive treatments, and medications to regulate hormone levels. It is important for patients to work closely with their healthcare team to develop a personalized treatment plan that addresses their specific cognitive symptoms and needs.

In addition to medical interventions, patients may also benefit from support resources that can help them cope with the cognitive challenges of living with a pituitary tumor. Support groups, counseling services, and educational materials can provide valuable information and emotional support to patients as they navigate the journey of diagnosis, treatment, and recovery. By staying informed and seeking appropriate care, patients can better manage cognitive changes and improve their overall quality of life.

Emotional and Psychological Effects

Navigating a diagnosis of a pituitary tumor can be overwhelming and emotionally taxing for patients. The uncertainty of the future, the potential impact on one's health and well-being, and the stress of managing symptoms can all contribute to feelings of anxiety, fear, and sadness. It is important for patients to acknowledge and address these emotional reactions in order to cope effectively with their diagnosis and treatment.

Treatment options for pituitary tumors can also have a significant impact on a patient's emotional and psychological well-being. The decision-making process can be daunting, as patients weigh the potential benefits and risks of surgery, radiation therapy, and medication. It is normal for patients to experience feelings of uncertainty, doubt, and fear as they navigate these choices. Seeking support from healthcare providers, loved ones, and support groups can help patients feel more confident in their treatment decisions.

Managing symptoms of pituitary tumors, such as headaches, vision changes, and hormonal imbalances, can take a toll on a patient's mental health. Chronic pain, fatigue, and changes in mood can all contribute to feelings of frustration, sadness, and isolation. It is important for patients to communicate openly with their healthcare team about their symptoms and seek appropriate treatment to improve their quality of life.

Surgical interventions for pituitary tumors can also have emotional and psychological effects on patients. The prospect of undergoing surgery, the recovery process, and the potential long-term effects of treatment can all be sources of stress and anxiety. Patients may benefit from counseling, support groups, and other resources to help them cope with the emotional challenges of surgery and recovery.

In conclusion, it is important for patients with pituitary tumors to recognize and address the emotional and psychological effects of their diagnosis and treatment. Seeking support from healthcare providers, loved ones, and support groups can help patients cope with the challenges of navigating their diagnosis, managing symptoms, and undergoing treatment. By taking steps to prioritize their mental health and well-being, patients can improve their quality of life and enhance their ability to cope with the emotional challenges of living with a pituitary tumor.

Chapter 5: Surgical Interventions for Pituitary Tumors

Transsphenoidal Surgery

Transsphenoidal surgery is a common surgical intervention used to treat pituitary tumors. This procedure involves accessing the pituitary gland through the nasal passages and sphenoid sinus, allowing for the removal of the tumor without the need for a traditional craniotomy. Transsphenoidal surgery is often considered the gold standard for treating pituitary tumors, as it is minimally invasive and has a high success rate.

During transsphenoidal surgery, a neurosurgeon will use specialized instruments to navigate through the nasal passages and sphenoid sinus to reach the pituitary gland. Once the tumor is located, the surgeon will carefully remove it, taking care to preserve surrounding healthy tissue. In some cases, the surgeon may also need to repair the sella turcica, the bony structure that houses the pituitary gland, to prevent cerebrospinal fluid leaks.

After transsphenoidal surgery, patients may experience some discomfort, such as nasal congestion, headaches, or a sore throat. However, these symptoms are typically mild and can be managed with medication. Most patients are able to go home within a few days of surgery and can return to their normal activities within a few weeks.

It is important for patients undergoing transsphenoidal surgery to follow their healthcare provider's instructions for post-operative care, including taking any prescribed medications and attending follow-up appointments. These appointments are crucial for monitoring recovery and ensuring that the tumor has been successfully removed. Patients should also be aware of potential complications, such as infection or hormonal imbalances, and report any unusual symptoms to their healthcare provider immediately.

Overall, transsphenoidal surgery is an effective treatment option for pituitary tumors, with a high success rate and low risk of complications. By understanding the process of transsphenoidal surgery and following post-operative care instructions, patients can navigate their diagnosis and treatment with confidence. If you have any questions or concerns about transsphenoidal surgery, be sure to discuss them with your healthcare provider.

Craniotomy

Craniotomy is a surgical procedure often used in the treatment of pituitary tumors. During a craniotomy, a neurosurgeon makes an incision in the scalp and removes a portion of the skull to access the brain. This allows the surgeon to carefully remove the tumor without causing damage to surrounding brain tissue. Craniotomies are typically performed under general anesthesia and may require a hospital stay of several days for recovery.

One of the key benefits of craniotomy for pituitary tumors is the ability to achieve a complete removal of the tumor. This can help to alleviate symptoms caused by the tumor, such as headaches, vision problems, and hormonal imbalances. In some cases, a craniotomy may also be used to take a biopsy of the tumor for further analysis to determine the best course of treatment.

While craniotomy is an effective treatment option for pituitary tumors, it does come with risks and potential complications. These can include infection, bleeding, and damage to surrounding brain tissue. It is important for patients to discuss the potential risks and benefits of craniotomy with their healthcare team to make an informed decision about their treatment plan.

After a craniotomy for a pituitary tumor, patients may experience some side effects such as headache, fatigue, and changes in hormone levels. It is important to follow post-operative care instructions provided by your healthcare team to help facilitate a smooth recovery. Regular follow-up appointments will also be necessary to monitor for any signs of tumor recurrence or other complications.

Overall, craniotomy can be an effective surgical intervention for pituitary tumors, but it is important for patients to weigh the potential risks and benefits before proceeding with this treatment option. Your healthcare team will work closely with you to provide support and guidance throughout the treatment process, and to help you navigate the complexities of living with a pituitary tumor.

Endoscopic Surgery

Endoscopic surgery is a minimally invasive surgical technique that is commonly used in the treatment of pituitary tumors. This approach involves the use of a thin, flexible tube with a camera and light at the end, allowing the surgeon to visualize the tumor and surrounding structures without the need for large incisions. Patients undergoing endoscopic surgery typically experience less pain, shorter hospital stays, and faster recovery times compared to traditional open surgery.

During endoscopic surgery for pituitary tumors, the surgeon will make a small incision in the nasal cavity or upper lip to access the tumor through the natural openings of the skull. The endoscope is then inserted through this opening, providing a clear view of the tumor and allowing for precise removal or destruction of the abnormal tissue. This targeted approach minimizes damage to healthy surrounding tissue, reducing the risk of complications and improving outcomes for patients.

Endoscopic surgery is often recommended for patients with pituitary tumors that are small to medium in size and located in the front of the pituitary gland. This technique is particularly effective for removing non-functioning tumors or those that produce excess hormones, helping to alleviate symptoms such as headaches, vision changes, and hormonal imbalances. In some cases, endoscopic surgery may be combined with other treatment modalities, such as radiation therapy or medication, to achieve the best possible outcome for the patient.

After endoscopic surgery for a pituitary tumor, patients can expect to be closely monitored by their healthcare team to ensure proper healing and recovery. Long-term follow-up care may include regular imaging studies to monitor for tumor recurrence, hormone level testing to assess pituitary function, and ongoing symptom management. It is important for patients to communicate openly with their healthcare providers about any concerns or changes in their condition to optimize their long-term health and well-being.

For patients undergoing endoscopic surgery for a pituitary tumor, it is essential to have a strong support system in place to help navigate the diagnosis, treatment, and recovery process. Support resources such as patient advocacy groups, online forums, and counseling services can provide valuable information and emotional support for individuals and their families. By actively engaging in their care and seeking out appropriate support, patients with pituitary tumors can effectively manage their condition and improve their overall quality of life.

Complications and Risks

When dealing with pituitary tumors, it is important to be aware of the potential complications and risks that may arise throughout the diagnosis and treatment process. While pituitary tumors are generally considered benign, they can still cause serious health issues if left untreated or if complications arise during treatment. It is essential for patients to understand these potential risks in order to make informed decisions about their care.

One of the primary complications of pituitary tumors is the impact they can have on hormone production and regulation within the body. Depending on the type of tumor and its location within the pituitary gland, patients may experience hormonal imbalances that can lead to a variety of symptoms, including fatigue, weight gain or loss, mood changes, and fertility issues. These hormonal imbalances can be challenging to manage and may require ongoing treatment to maintain optimal health.

Surgical interventions for pituitary tumors also come with inherent risks, such as bleeding, infection, and damage to surrounding structures in the brain. While these risks are relatively low, it is important for patients to discuss them with their healthcare team and weigh the potential benefits of surgery against the potential risks. Additionally, long-term effects of pituitary tumor surgery, such as changes in hormone levels or vision problems, should be considered when making treatment decisions.

Non-invasive treatment methods, such as medication or radiation therapy, also carry their own risks and potential complications. For example, certain medications used to treat pituitary tumors may have side effects that can impact a patient's quality of life. Radiation therapy, while effective in shrinking tumors, can also cause damage to surrounding tissues and organs. Patients should be aware of these potential risks and work closely with their healthcare team to monitor and manage any complications that may arise.

In addition to the physical complications of pituitary tumors and their treatment, patients may also experience emotional and psychological challenges. The impact of a pituitary tumor diagnosis on mental health and well-being should not be overlooked, as patients may experience anxiety, depression, or feelings of isolation. It is important for patients to seek support from healthcare providers, mental health professionals, and support resources to address these issues and maintain a positive outlook throughout their treatment journey.

Recovery and Rehabilitation

After undergoing treatment for a pituitary tumor, it is important for patients to focus on their recovery and rehabilitation process. This phase is crucial in ensuring a successful outcome and maintaining overall health and well-being. Recovery may vary depending on the type of treatment received, but there are general guidelines that can help patients navigate this period effectively.

One of the key aspects of recovery is managing symptoms of pituitary tumors. This may involve taking medications to regulate hormone levels, as well as addressing any physical or emotional side effects of treatment. It is important for patients to communicate openly with their healthcare team about any symptoms they may be experiencing, as they can provide guidance on how to best manage them.

Surgical interventions for pituitary tumors may require a longer recovery period compared to non-invasive treatment methods. Patients who undergo surgery should follow their healthcare team's post-operative instructions carefully to promote healing and prevent complications. It is also important for patients to attend follow-up appointments to monitor their progress and address any concerns that may arise during the recovery process.

In addition to physical recovery, patients should also focus on rehabilitation to address any hormonal imbalances caused by pituitary tumors. This may involve ongoing hormone replacement therapy or other treatments to help restore hormonal balance and improve overall well-being. Patients should work closely with their healthcare team to develop a personalized rehabilitation plan that meets their individual needs.

Throughout the recovery and rehabilitation process, patients may experience a range of emotions related to their diagnosis and treatment. It is important for patients to seek support from loved ones, as well as from support resources for patients with pituitary tumors. These resources can provide valuable information, guidance, and emotional support to help patients navigate the challenges of recovery and maintain their mental health and well-being. By focusing on recovery and rehabilitation, patients can take an active role in their healing journey and work towards a positive outcome.

Chapter 6: Non-Invasive Treatment Methods for Pituitary Tumors

Stereotactic Radiosurgery

Stereotactic radiosurgery is a non-invasive treatment option for patients with pituitary tumors. This advanced technique delivers targeted radiation to the tumor, while minimizing damage to surrounding healthy tissue. Stereotactic radiosurgery is often used in cases where surgery is not possible or has not been successful in completely removing the tumor. This treatment method can help to shrink the tumor and reduce symptoms caused by the tumor's growth.

During stereotactic radiosurgery, patients are fitted with a specialized head frame to ensure precise delivery of radiation to the tumor. The procedure is typically performed on an outpatient basis and does not require a hospital stay. Most patients experience minimal discomfort during the treatment and are able to resume their normal activities shortly afterwards. It is important for patients to follow their healthcare provider's instructions for follow-up care and monitoring after stereotactic radiosurgery.

One of the benefits of stereotactic radiosurgery is its ability to target tumors located in critical or hard-to-reach areas of the brain, such as the pituitary gland. This treatment method can be particularly effective for patients with pituitary tumors that are small in size or are not causing significant symptoms. Stereotactic radiosurgery may also be used in combination with other treatment modalities, such as medication or traditional radiation therapy, to provide comprehensive care for patients with pituitary tumors.

While stereotactic radiosurgery is generally well-tolerated, some patients may experience side effects such as fatigue, headache, or nausea. These side effects are typically mild and temporary, and can be managed with medication or other supportive measures. It is important for patients to communicate any concerns or symptoms to their healthcare provider, so that appropriate care can be provided. Overall, stereotactic radiosurgery is a valuable treatment option for patients with pituitary tumors, offering a minimally invasive approach to tumor management.

In conclusion, stereotactic radiosurgery is a safe and effective treatment option for patients with pituitary tumors. This non-invasive technique can help to reduce the size of the tumor and alleviate symptoms, improving the overall quality of life for patients. By working closely with a multidisciplinary healthcare team, patients can navigate their diagnosis and treatment plan with confidence. It is important for patients to stay informed about their condition and treatment options, and to seek support from healthcare providers and support resources as needed. With proper care and management, patients with pituitary tumors can live well and thrive in their journey towards health and well-being.

Gamma Knife Therapy

Gamma Knife therapy is a non-invasive treatment option for patients with pituitary tumors that utilizes highly focused radiation beams to target and destroy tumor cells. This innovative approach offers many benefits, including minimal side effects, precise targeting of the tumor, and the ability to spare surrounding healthy tissue. Gamma Knife therapy is particularly well-suited for patients who may not be candidates for traditional surgery or who prefer a less invasive treatment option.

During Gamma Knife therapy, patients are fitted with a specialized head frame to ensure accurate targeting of the radiation beams. The treatment itself is painless and typically lasts between 15 minutes to a few hours, depending on the size and location of the tumor. Patients may experience mild side effects such as headache or nausea, but these are usually temporary and can be managed with medication.

One of the key advantages of Gamma Knife therapy is its ability to deliver high doses of radiation to the tumor while minimizing exposure to surrounding healthy tissue. This targeted approach helps to reduce the risk of damage to critical structures in the brain and can result in improved outcomes for patients. Additionally, Gamma Knife therapy can be used in combination with other treatments such as surgery or medication to provide a comprehensive approach to managing pituitary tumors.

After undergoing Gamma Knife therapy, patients will typically have follow-up appointments to monitor their progress and assess the effectiveness of the treatment. It is important for patients to communicate any changes in symptoms or side effects to their healthcare team so that appropriate adjustments can be made to their treatment plan. In some cases, additional rounds of Gamma Knife therapy may be recommended to further target residual tumor cells or prevent recurrence.

Overall, Gamma Knife therapy is a valuable treatment option for patients with pituitary tumors, offering a safe and effective alternative to traditional surgery. By working closely with their healthcare team and staying informed about their condition, patients can navigate the complexities of pituitary tumor treatment with confidence and achieve the best possible outcomes for their health and well-being.

CyberKnife Radiosurgery

CyberKnife Radiosurgery is a non-invasive treatment option for patients with pituitary tumors, offering a precise and targeted approach to tumor removal. This cutting-edge technology delivers high doses of radiation to the tumor while minimizing exposure to surrounding healthy tissue. CyberKnife Radiosurgery is particularly beneficial for patients who may not be candidates for traditional surgery due to the location or size of the tumor.

One of the key advantages of CyberKnife Radiosurgery is its ability to deliver treatment in a shorter timeframe compared to conventional radiation therapy. This can result in fewer treatment sessions and reduced overall treatment duration, leading to improved patient convenience and comfort. Additionally, CyberKnife Radiosurgery has been shown to be effective in controlling the growth of pituitary tumors and relieving symptoms associated with hormonal imbalances.

Patients undergoing CyberKnife Radiosurgery can expect minimal side effects, with most experiencing little to no discomfort during treatment. The precise targeting of the radiation allows for a high level of accuracy, reducing the risk of damage to nearby structures and organs. Following treatment, patients can typically resume their normal activities without the need for an extended recovery period.

It is important for patients considering CyberKnife Radiosurgery to have a thorough discussion with their healthcare team about the potential benefits and risks of this treatment option. While CyberKnife Radiosurgery is generally well-tolerated, some patients may experience temporary side effects such as fatigue or mild headaches. Close monitoring and follow-up care are essential to ensure the best possible outcomes for patients undergoing this innovative treatment for pituitary tumors.

In conclusion, CyberKnife Radiosurgery offers a safe and effective treatment option for patients with pituitary tumors, providing targeted therapy with minimal side effects. By working closely with a multidisciplinary team of healthcare professionals, patients can make informed decisions about their treatment plan and feel confident in the care they receive. With advancements in technology and treatment options, patients with pituitary tumors can look forward to improved outcomes and a better quality of life.

Proton Therapy

Proton therapy is a type of radiation therapy that is used to treat pituitary tumors. This form of treatment delivers high-energy protons directly to the tumor site, minimizing damage to surrounding healthy tissue. Proton therapy is particularly beneficial for patients with pituitary tumors located close to critical structures such as the optic nerves or brainstem, where preserving function is essential.

One of the key advantages of proton therapy is its ability to precisely target the tumor while sparing nearby organs from unnecessary radiation exposure. This targeted approach reduces the risk of side effects commonly associated with traditional radiation therapy, such as damage to the pituitary gland or surrounding brain tissue. As a result, patients undergoing proton therapy may experience fewer long-term complications and enjoy a better quality of life post-treatment.

Patients considering proton therapy for pituitary tumors should consult with a multidisciplinary team of healthcare providers to determine if this treatment option is appropriate for their specific case. The decision to pursue proton therapy should take into account factors such as tumor size, location, and overall health status. Additionally, patients should discuss the potential benefits and risks of proton therapy with their healthcare team to make an informed decision about their treatment plan.

During proton therapy, patients will undergo a series of treatment sessions over a period of several weeks. Each session typically lasts only a few minutes, during which time the patient will lie comfortably on a treatment table while the proton beam is delivered to the tumor site. Most patients tolerate proton therapy well, experiencing minimal discomfort or side effects. After completing treatment, patients will undergo regular follow-up appointments to monitor their progress and assess the effectiveness of proton therapy in controlling the tumor.

In conclusion, proton therapy is a valuable treatment option for patients with pituitary tumors, offering a targeted approach to radiation therapy that minimizes damage to surrounding healthy tissue. By working closely with their healthcare team to explore all available treatment options, patients can make informed decisions about their care and improve their chances for a successful outcome. With proper guidance and support, patients can navigate the complexities of pituitary tumor treatment and achieve optimal health and well-being.

Radiofrequency Ablation

Radiofrequency ablation is a minimally invasive procedure that may be used to treat pituitary tumors in certain cases. During this procedure, a special needle is inserted into the tumor under the guidance of imaging techniques such as MRI or CT scans. Once the needle is in place, high-frequency electrical currents are used to heat and destroy the tumor tissue. Radiofrequency ablation is typically performed by an interventional radiologist and may be done on an outpatient basis.

One of the benefits of radiofrequency ablation is that it can be an effective treatment option for patients who are not good candidates for surgery or who prefer a less invasive approach. This procedure is also associated with fewer risks and complications compared to traditional surgical methods. Additionally, radiofrequency ablation may result in shorter recovery times and less post-operative discomfort for patients.

It is important to note that radiofrequency ablation may not be suitable for all types of pituitary tumors. Your healthcare provider will determine if this treatment option is appropriate for your specific situation based on factors such as the size and location of the tumor, as well as your overall health and medical history. It is essential to have a thorough discussion with your healthcare team to fully understand the potential benefits and risks of radiofrequency ablation before proceeding with this treatment.

As with any medical procedure, there are potential risks and side effects associated with radiofrequency ablation. These may include temporary pain or discomfort at the site of the procedure, as well as the possibility of bleeding, infection, or damage to surrounding tissues. Your healthcare provider will discuss these risks with you in detail and help you make an informed decision about whether radiofrequency ablation is the right choice for you.

In conclusion, radiofrequency ablation is a non-invasive treatment method that may be used to target and destroy pituitary tumors. This procedure offers certain advantages over traditional surgical interventions, such as a shorter recovery time and fewer complications. However, it is essential to consult with your healthcare provider to determine if radiofrequency ablation is the most appropriate treatment option for your individual case. By working closely with your medical team, you can make informed decisions about managing your pituitary tumor and improving your overall health and well-being.

Chapter 7: Hormonal Imbalances Caused by Pituitary Tumors

Hypersecretion Disorders

Hypersecretion disorders refer to conditions in which the pituitary gland produces an excess amount of hormones. This can be caused by a pituitary tumor, which disrupts the normal functioning of the gland and leads to overproduction of hormones. Common hypersecretion disorders associated with pituitary tumors include acromegaly, Cushing's disease, and hyperprolactinemia. These disorders can have a significant impact on the body's hormonal balance and overall health.

Patients with hypersecretion disorders may experience a range of symptoms, depending on the specific hormones that are being overproduced. For example, individuals with acromegaly may notice changes in their appearance, such as enlarged hands and feet, while those with Cushing's disease may experience weight gain, high blood pressure, and mood swings. Hyperprolactinemia, on the other hand, can lead to irregular menstrual periods, infertility, and breast milk production in both men and women.

Treatment options for hypersecretion disorders caused by pituitary tumors typically focus on reducing the production of excess hormones. This may involve medications to suppress hormone production, radiation therapy to shrink the tumor, or surgical removal of the tumor. The choice of treatment will depend on the type and size of the tumor, as well as the patient's overall health and preferences.

In some cases, managing the symptoms of hypersecretion disorders may also involve addressing hormonal imbalances caused by the pituitary tumor. This may include hormone replacement therapy to restore normal hormone levels and alleviate symptoms such as fatigue, weight gain, and mood changes. It is important for patients to work closely with their healthcare team to develop a comprehensive treatment plan that addresses both the tumor itself and its effects on the body.

Overall, hypersecretion disorders associated with pituitary tumors can have a significant impact on a patient's physical and emotional well-being. It is important for patients to seek support from healthcare providers, support groups, and other resources to help them navigate their diagnosis and treatment. By working closely with their healthcare team and staying informed about their condition, patients can better manage their symptoms, improve their quality of life, and reduce the risk of tumor recurrence.

Hyposecretion Disorders

Hyposecretion disorders refer to conditions where the pituitary gland produces insufficient amounts of hormones, leading to various health problems. Patients with hyposecretion disorders may experience symptoms such as fatigue, weight gain, low blood pressure, and decreased libido. These disorders can be caused by pituitary tumors that disrupt the normal functioning of the gland. It is essential for patients to understand the implications of hyposecretion disorders and seek appropriate treatment to manage their symptoms effectively.

Treatment options for hyposecretion disorders caused by pituitary tumors may include hormone replacement therapy to restore hormone levels to normal. This can help alleviate symptoms and improve the patient's overall quality of life. In some cases, surgical intervention may be necessary to remove the tumor and restore proper hormone production. It is important for patients to work closely with their healthcare providers to determine the best course of treatment for their specific condition.

Managing the symptoms of hyposecretion disorders can be challenging, but there are ways to improve quality of life. Patients should focus on maintaining a healthy lifestyle, including regular exercise, balanced nutrition, and adequate rest. It is also important to follow the treatment plan prescribed by healthcare providers and attend regular follow-up appointments to monitor hormone levels and adjust treatment as needed. By taking an active role in their healthcare, patients can effectively manage the symptoms of hyposecretion disorders and improve their overall well-being.

Surgical interventions for hyposecretion disorders caused by pituitary tumors may involve transsphenoidal surgery, a minimally invasive procedure that removes the tumor through the nasal cavity. This approach can help preserve normal pituitary function and reduce the risk of complications. Patients undergoing surgery should be prepared for a period of recovery and follow-up care to monitor hormone levels and ensure the success of the procedure. It is important for patients to discuss the risks and benefits of surgical intervention with their healthcare team and make informed decisions about their treatment.

Non-invasive treatment methods, such as radiation therapy or medication, may also be used to manage hyposecretion disorders caused by pituitary tumors. These approaches can help shrink the tumor and restore normal hormone production without the need for surgery. Patients should work closely with their healthcare providers to determine the most appropriate treatment approach based on their individual needs and preferences. By exploring all available options and staying informed about their condition, patients can effectively manage hyposecretion disorders and improve their overall health and well-being.

Hormone Replacement Therapy

Hormone replacement therapy is often a crucial aspect of treatment for patients with pituitary tumors, as these tumors can disrupt the normal production of hormones by the pituitary gland. The pituitary gland plays a key role in regulating various hormones in the body, so when a tumor develops in this gland, it can lead to hormonal imbalances that affect multiple bodily functions. Hormone replacement therapy is used to restore these hormone levels to normal, helping patients manage their symptoms and improve their overall quality of life.

There are different types of hormone replacement therapy available, depending on the specific hormones that are affected by the pituitary tumor. For example, patients with low levels of thyroid hormone may be prescribed thyroid hormone replacement therapy, while those with low levels of cortisol may require cortisol replacement therapy. It is important for patients to work closely with their healthcare providers to determine the appropriate type and dosage of hormone replacement therapy for their individual needs.

Hormone replacement therapy can help alleviate a wide range of symptoms associated with pituitary tumors, such as fatigue, weight gain, mood changes, and sexual dysfunction. By restoring hormone levels to normal, patients may experience improvements in their energy levels, mood, and overall sense of well-being. It is important for patients to communicate openly with their healthcare providers about any changes or improvements they may experience while undergoing hormone replacement therapy.

In addition to hormone replacement therapy, patients with pituitary tumors may also require other treatments such as surgery, radiation therapy, or medication. These treatments are often used in combination to effectively manage the tumor and its associated symptoms. It is important for patients to follow their treatment plan closely and attend regular follow-up appointments to monitor their progress and adjust their treatment as needed.

Overall, hormone replacement therapy is an important component of treatment for patients with pituitary tumors. By restoring hormone levels to normal, patients can better manage their symptoms and improve their quality of life. It is essential for patients to work closely with their healthcare providers to ensure they are receiving the appropriate type and dosage of hormone replacement therapy for their individual needs.

Monitoring and Management

Monitoring and managing pituitary tumors are crucial aspects of treatment that require ongoing attention and care. Patients with pituitary tumors must work closely with their healthcare team to ensure that their condition is properly monitored and any changes in symptoms or tumor growth are addressed promptly. Regular follow-up appointments, imaging studies, and hormonal tests are essential for tracking the progress of the tumor and evaluating the effectiveness of treatment.

Treatment options for pituitary tumors vary depending on the type and size of the tumor, as well as the individual patient's overall health and preferences. Surgical intervention may be recommended to remove the tumor, especially if it is causing symptoms or affecting hormone production. Non-invasive treatment methods, such as radiation therapy or medication, may also be used to manage pituitary tumors and help control symptoms.

Managing symptoms of pituitary tumors can be challenging, as they can vary widely depending on the type of tumor and the hormones it affects. Patients may experience headaches, vision changes, hormonal imbalances, and other symptoms that can significantly impact their quality of life. Working closely with healthcare providers to manage these symptoms through medications, lifestyle changes, and other interventions is essential for improving overall well-being.

Surgical interventions for pituitary tumors may be necessary in some cases to remove the tumor and alleviate symptoms. Transsphenoidal surgery is a common approach for removing pituitary tumors, as it involves accessing the tumor through the nasal cavity and does not require a craniotomy. Patients undergoing surgery should be aware of the potential risks and complications associated with the procedure, as well as the expected recovery time and follow-up care.

Monitoring hormone levels and managing hormonal imbalances caused by pituitary tumors are important aspects of treatment that require ongoing attention and care. Patients may need to take hormone replacement therapy or other medications to help regulate hormone levels and alleviate symptoms. Genetic factors related to pituitary tumors may also play a role in treatment decisions, as some patients may have a higher risk of developing pituitary tumors due to inherited genetic mutations. Working closely with genetic counselors and other specialists can help patients better understand their risk factors and make informed decisions about their treatment plan.

Long-Term Effects

Long-term effects of pituitary tumor surgery can vary depending on the specific type of tumor, the location of the tumor, and the individual patient's overall health. While many patients experience positive outcomes following surgery, it is important to be aware of potential long-term effects that may impact your quality of life. These effects can include hormonal imbalances, changes in vision, cognitive changes, and emotional challenges.

One common long-term effect of pituitary tumor surgery is the development of hormonal imbalances. This can occur when the surgery disrupts the normal function of the pituitary gland, leading to deficiencies or excesses of certain hormones. It is important for patients to work closely with their healthcare team to monitor and manage these imbalances through hormone replacement therapy or other interventions to prevent complications.

Another potential long-term effect of pituitary tumor surgery is changes in vision. Depending on the location of the tumor and the extent of the surgery, patients may experience visual disturbances such as double vision, blurry vision, or decreased peripheral vision. It is crucial for patients to have regular follow-up appointments with their ophthalmologist to monitor any changes in vision and address any concerns promptly.

Cognitive changes, such as memory problems or difficulty concentrating, can also be a long-term effect of pituitary tumor surgery. These changes may be related to the disruption of hormone levels or the stress of undergoing surgery. Patients experiencing cognitive changes should communicate with their healthcare team to develop strategies to improve cognitive function and overall well-being.

Emotional challenges, such as anxiety, depression, or mood swings, can also arise as a long-term effect of pituitary tumor surgery. It is important for patients to seek support from mental health professionals, support groups, or other resources to address these emotional challenges and maintain their mental health and well-being. By staying informed, proactive, and engaged in their care, patients can navigate the long-term effects of pituitary tumor surgery and optimize their overall quality of life.

Chapter 8: Genetic Factors Related to Pituitary Tumors

Familial Pituitary Tumor Syndromes

Familial Pituitary Tumor Syndromes are a rare but important aspect of pituitary tumor diagnosis and treatment. In some cases, pituitary tumors can run in families, indicating a genetic predisposition to these types of tumors. Understanding the genetic factors related to pituitary tumors can help patients and their healthcare providers determine the best course of action for diagnosis, treatment, and long-term management.

When it comes to Familial Pituitary Tumor Syndromes, it is crucial for patients to undergo genetic testing to identify any mutations or inherited genetic factors that may be contributing to the development of pituitary tumors. This information can help healthcare providers tailor treatment plans and surveillance strategies to address the specific needs of patients with familial predispositions to pituitary tumors.

Patients with Familial Pituitary Tumor Syndromes may require more frequent screening and monitoring to detect tumors at an earlier stage when they are more easily treatable. Additionally, genetic counseling may be recommended to help patients and their families understand their risk factors and make informed decisions about their healthcare.

In cases where surgical intervention is necessary for pituitary tumors associated with Familial Pituitary Tumor Syndromes, patients may need to consider the long-term effects of surgery on hormonal balance and overall health. It is important for patients to work closely with their healthcare team to manage any hormonal imbalances that may arise as a result of surgery or other treatment modalities.

While dealing with Familial Pituitary Tumor Syndromes can be challenging, there are support resources available to help patients navigate their diagnosis and treatment journey. By staying informed, proactive, and in communication with their healthcare providers, patients can take control of their health and well-being in the face of pituitary tumors and genetic predispositions.

Genetic Testing and Counseling

Genetic testing and counseling play a crucial role in understanding the underlying factors that may contribute to the development of pituitary tumors. By undergoing genetic testing, patients can gain valuable insights into their genetic makeup and any potential predispositions to developing pituitary tumors. This information can help healthcare providers tailor treatment plans and provide personalized care to address the specific needs of each patient.

Genetic testing can also help identify any hereditary factors that may increase the risk of developing pituitary tumors. In some cases, certain genetic mutations or syndromes may be linked to an increased likelihood of developing these tumors. By identifying these genetic factors early on, patients and their healthcare providers can take proactive steps to monitor for potential tumor growth and implement preventive measures to reduce the risk of tumor development.

Genetic counseling is an essential component of the genetic testing process, providing patients with the opportunity to discuss their test results, understand the implications of any genetic findings, and explore their options for managing their risk of developing pituitary tumors. Genetic counselors are trained to provide support, guidance, and education to patients and their families, helping them make informed decisions about their healthcare and genetic testing options.

For patients with a family history of pituitary tumors or other genetic risk factors, genetic counseling can be particularly valuable in helping them navigate their treatment options and make informed decisions about their healthcare. Genetic counselors can provide patients with information on the latest advancements in genetic testing, treatment options, and preventive measures, empowering them to take an active role in managing their health and well-being.

Overall, genetic testing and counseling can play a pivotal role in the management and treatment of pituitary tumors, providing patients with valuable insights into their genetic makeup and any potential risk factors for tumor development. By working closely with their healthcare providers and genetic counselors, patients can take proactive steps to monitor for tumor growth, manage their risk factors, and make informed decisions about their healthcare.

Risk Assessment and Screening

Risk assessment and screening are essential components in the diagnosis and treatment of pituitary tumors. As a patient navigating the complexities of this condition, it is important to understand the various factors that can contribute to the development and progression of these tumors. By conducting a thorough risk assessment, healthcare providers can determine the likelihood of a pituitary tumor and tailor treatment options accordingly.

Screening for pituitary tumors typically involves a combination of medical history review, physical examination, and imaging tests such as MRI or CT scans. These diagnostic tools help healthcare providers identify the location, size, and characteristics of the tumor, which are crucial in determining the most appropriate treatment approach. It is important for patients to actively participate in the screening process by providing accurate and detailed information about their symptoms, medical history, and any genetic predispositions that may be relevant.

In addition to physical screening, healthcare providers may also assess the risk of hormonal imbalances caused by pituitary tumors. Hormonal imbalances can manifest in a variety of ways, including changes in weight, mood, energy levels, and reproductive health. By closely monitoring hormone levels and symptoms, healthcare providers can better understand the impact of the tumor on the body and develop targeted treatment plans to address these imbalances.

Genetic factors play a significant role in the development of pituitary tumors, with certain gene mutations increasing the risk of tumor formation. Patients with a family history of pituitary tumors or genetic syndromes associated with these tumors may be at higher risk and should undergo regular screening to detect any abnormalities at an early stage. Understanding these genetic factors can help patients and healthcare providers make informed decisions about treatment and monitoring strategies.

In conclusion, risk assessment and screening are critical components in the management of pituitary tumors. By actively participating in the screening process and providing accurate information to healthcare providers, patients can receive timely and appropriate treatment for their condition. Genetic factors, hormonal imbalances, and long-term effects of surgery are all important considerations in the risk assessment process, and patients should work closely with their healthcare team to navigate these complexities and optimize their treatment outcomes.

Prevention Strategies

Preventing the recurrence of pituitary tumors is a crucial aspect of managing this condition. While there is no definitive way to completely prevent the development of pituitary tumors, there are several strategies that may help reduce the risk of recurrence. One of the most important prevention strategies is regular monitoring and follow-up care with your healthcare provider. By staying vigilant and monitoring your symptoms closely, you and your healthcare team can catch any potential recurrence early and take appropriate action.

Another key prevention strategy is to adhere to your prescribed treatment plan. Whether you undergo surgery, radiation therapy, or other forms of treatment, it is essential to follow your healthcare provider's recommendations and attend all follow-up appointments. By staying proactive and engaged in your treatment plan, you can help prevent the recurrence of pituitary tumors and manage any potential complications that may arise.

Maintaining a healthy lifestyle is also important for preventing the recurrence of pituitary tumors. Eating a balanced diet, getting regular exercise, and managing stress can all contribute to overall well-being and may help reduce the risk of tumor recurrence. Additionally, avoiding tobacco and excessive alcohol consumption can further lower your risk of developing complications related to pituitary tumors.

It is also essential to be aware of any genetic factors that may play a role in the development of pituitary tumors. If you have a family history of pituitary tumors or other related conditions, be sure to discuss this with your healthcare provider. Genetic counseling may be recommended to assess your risk and determine appropriate prevention strategies.

In conclusion, while there is no foolproof way to prevent the development or recurrence of pituitary tumors, there are several strategies that can help lower your risk and manage this condition effectively. By staying proactive, adhering to your treatment plan, maintaining a healthy lifestyle, and being aware of any genetic factors, you can take control of your health and work towards preventing the recurrence of pituitary tumors. Remember, you are not alone in this journey – your healthcare team is here to support you every step of the way.

Family Planning Considerations

Family planning considerations are an important aspect to consider for patients diagnosed with pituitary tumors. These tumors can have an impact on fertility and hormonal balance, which may affect a patient's ability to conceive or carry a pregnancy to full term. It is crucial for patients to discuss their family planning goals with their healthcare team to ensure that they receive appropriate guidance and support.

Patients with pituitary tumors may experience hormonal imbalances that can affect their reproductive health. For women, irregular menstrual cycles, ovulation disorders, and infertility may be common concerns. Men may experience decreased libido, erectile dysfunction, and decreased sperm production. These issues can make it difficult for patients to conceive naturally, and they may need to explore alternative options such as assisted reproductive technologies.

When considering family planning options, patients with pituitary tumors should work closely with their healthcare team to develop a personalized plan that takes into account their specific medical needs and treatment goals. Depending on the type and size of the tumor, as well as the treatment options chosen, patients may need to delay or modify their plans for starting a family. It is important to have open and honest discussions with healthcare providers to ensure that all aspects of family planning are considered.

Patients who have undergone surgery or other treatments for pituitary tumors should be aware of the potential impact on their fertility and hormonal function. Some treatments, such as radiation therapy or certain medications, may cause temporary or permanent damage to the pituitary gland, which can affect fertility. It is important to discuss these potential risks with healthcare providers and to explore options for preserving fertility before undergoing treatment.

In conclusion, family planning considerations are an important aspect of care for patients with pituitary tumors. By working closely with healthcare providers to develop a personalized plan that takes into account their specific medical needs and treatment goals, patients can make informed decisions about their reproductive health. It is important to have open and honest discussions with healthcare providers to ensure that all aspects of family planning are considered and that patients receive the support and guidance they need.

Chapter 9: Long-Term Effects of Pituitary Tumor Surgery

Pituitary Dysfunction

Pituitary dysfunction is a common issue that can arise as a result of pituitary tumors. The pituitary gland plays a crucial role in regulating various hormones in the body, so when it is not functioning properly due to a tumor, it can lead to a range of symptoms and complications. Understanding how pituitary dysfunction can impact your health is essential for navigating the diagnosis and treatment of pituitary tumors.

Treatment options for pituitary tumors vary depending on the size and location of the tumor, as well as the symptoms it is causing. In some cases, surgical intervention may be necessary to remove the tumor and alleviate pressure on the surrounding structures. However, there are also non-invasive treatment methods available, such as medication or radiation therapy, that can help shrink the tumor and control hormone levels.

Managing symptoms of pituitary tumors is an important aspect of treatment for patients. Hormonal imbalances caused by pituitary tumors can lead to a range of symptoms, including fatigue, weight gain, mood changes, and fertility issues. It is crucial to work closely with your healthcare team to address these symptoms and develop a personalized treatment plan to improve your quality of life.

Surgical interventions for pituitary tumors carry their own set of risks and potential complications. It is important to discuss these with your healthcare team and understand the long-term effects of pituitary tumor surgery. Additionally, genetic factors may play a role in the development of pituitary tumors, so it is important to consider your family history and any predisposing factors.

Support resources for patients with pituitary tumors are available to help navigate the challenges of diagnosis, treatment, and recovery. These resources can provide emotional support, educational materials, and practical assistance to help you cope with the impact of pituitary tumors on your mental health and well-being. By staying informed and connected to your healthcare team and support network, you can better manage pituitary dysfunction and improve your overall quality of life.

Cognitive Impairment

"Cognitive Impairment"

Cognitive impairment refers to difficulties with memory, concentration, and other aspects of thinking that can result from a pituitary tumor. Patients with pituitary tumors may experience cognitive changes due to hormonal imbalances, pressure on the brain from the tumor, or side effects of treatment. It is important for patients to be aware of these potential challenges and to work with their healthcare team to address them.

Patients with pituitary tumors may experience difficulty with short-term memory, attention, and problem-solving abilities. These cognitive changes can have a significant impact on daily life, making it important to seek appropriate support and interventions. Cognitive impairment can also affect emotional well-being and overall quality of life, highlighting the importance of addressing these challenges in a comprehensive treatment plan.

Managing cognitive impairment in patients with pituitary tumors may involve a combination of strategies, including cognitive rehabilitation, medication management, and lifestyle modifications. Cognitive rehabilitation programs can help patients improve their memory, attention, and other cognitive skills through targeted exercises and therapies. Medications may also be prescribed to help manage cognitive symptoms, such as difficulties with concentration or mood changes.

In addition to cognitive rehabilitation and medication management, lifestyle modifications can also play a role in managing cognitive impairment in patients with pituitary tumors. These may include engaging in regular physical activity, maintaining a healthy diet, and practicing stress-reducing techniques such as mindfulness or relaxation exercises. By taking a comprehensive approach to managing cognitive impairment, patients can improve their overall quality of life and well-being.

Overall, cognitive impairment is a common challenge for patients with pituitary tumors, but it is important to remember that there are strategies and interventions available to help manage these symptoms. By working closely with their healthcare team and taking a proactive approach to addressing cognitive changes, patients can improve their cognitive function and overall quality of life. It is important for patients to seek support and resources to help navigate the challenges of cognitive impairment and to advocate for their own well-being throughout their treatment journey.

Neurological Complications

Neurological complications are a common concern for patients with pituitary tumors. These complications can arise due to the size and location of the tumor, as well as the pressure it exerts on surrounding brain structures. Some of the most common neurological complications associated with pituitary tumors include vision changes, headaches, and hormonal imbalances. It is important for patients to be aware of these potential complications and to work closely with their healthcare team to address them.

Vision changes are often one of the first signs of a pituitary tumor, as the tumor can press on the optic nerves and cause visual disturbances. Patients may experience blurry vision, double vision, or even loss of peripheral vision. It is crucial for patients to report any changes in vision to their healthcare provider promptly, as early intervention can help prevent permanent vision loss. Treatment options for vision changes caused by pituitary tumors may include surgery to remove the tumor or medication to reduce swelling and pressure on the optic nerves.

Headaches are another common neurological complication associated with pituitary tumors. These headaches can be severe and debilitating, impacting a patient's quality of life. Patients may also experience nausea, vomiting, and sensitivity to light. Managing headache symptoms may involve a combination of medication, lifestyle changes, and stress management techniques. It is essential for patients to communicate openly with their healthcare team about their symptoms and to work together to develop a personalized treatment plan.

Hormonal imbalances are another potential neurological complication of pituitary tumors. The pituitary gland plays a crucial role in regulating hormone levels in the body, so a tumor in this gland can disrupt the delicate balance of hormones. Patients may experience symptoms such as fatigue, weight gain, mood changes, and menstrual irregularities. Treatment for hormonal imbalances may involve medication, hormone replacement therapy, or surgery to remove the tumor. It is important for patients to undergo regular hormone level monitoring and to follow their healthcare provider's recommendations for managing these imbalances.

In conclusion, neurological complications are a significant concern for patients with pituitary tumors. It is essential for patients to be proactive in monitoring and addressing these complications to prevent long-term consequences. By working closely with their healthcare team and staying informed about potential symptoms and treatment options, patients can navigate the challenges of pituitary tumors with confidence and resilience.

Psychosocial Challenges

Living with a pituitary tumor can present a variety of psychosocial challenges for patients. The diagnosis of a pituitary tumor can be overwhelming and may lead to feelings of anxiety, fear, and uncertainty. Patients may struggle to come to terms with their diagnosis and may experience a range of emotions as they navigate the complexities of treatment options and managing symptoms.

It is important for patients to recognize that they are not alone in facing these challenges. Seeking support from healthcare providers, family members, and support groups can help patients cope with the emotional impact of living with a pituitary tumor. Talking openly about feelings and concerns can provide patients with a sense of relief and validation, and may help them develop coping strategies to address their psychosocial needs.

Managing the symptoms of a pituitary tumor can also have a significant impact on a patient's mental health and well-being. Hormonal imbalances caused by the tumor can lead to changes in mood, energy levels, and overall quality of life. Patients may experience fatigue, depression, and difficulty concentrating, which can further exacerbate the psychosocial challenges they face.

Surgical interventions for pituitary tumors can also have long-term effects on a patient's mental health. While surgery is often necessary to remove the tumor and alleviate symptoms, patients may experience emotional distress and anxiety related to the procedure and its outcomes. It is important for patients to have realistic expectations about the potential emotional impact of surgery and to seek support from healthcare providers and mental health professionals as needed.

In conclusion, it is essential for patients with pituitary tumors to address the psychosocial challenges they face in order to improve their overall well-being and quality of life. By seeking support, talking openly about feelings, and developing coping strategies, patients can navigate the emotional complexities of living with a pituitary tumor. Healthcare providers play a crucial role in helping patients address their psychosocial needs and should work collaboratively with patients to provide holistic care that addresses both the physical and emotional aspects of living with a pituitary tumor.

Survivorship Care Planning

Survivorship care planning is a crucial aspect of managing pituitary tumors and ensuring long-term health and well-being for patients. After undergoing treatment for a pituitary tumor, it is important to have a comprehensive plan in place to address ongoing medical needs, manage any lingering symptoms, and monitor for potential recurrence. This chapter will outline the key components of survivorship care planning and provide guidance for patients navigating life after treatment.

One of the first steps in survivorship care planning is establishing a follow-up schedule with your healthcare team. Regular check-ups and monitoring are essential to detect any signs of tumor recurrence or hormonal imbalances early on. Your healthcare provider will work with you to develop a personalized plan based on your specific needs and medical history. This may include regular imaging scans, blood tests, and hormonal assessments to ensure your health and well-being are being properly monitored.

In addition to medical follow-up, survivorship care planning may also involve addressing any lingering symptoms or side effects from treatment. This could include managing hormonal imbalances, addressing cognitive changes, or dealing with emotional distress related to your diagnosis and treatment. Your healthcare team can provide support and guidance on managing these symptoms and improving your overall quality of life.

Surgical interventions for pituitary tumors may have long-term effects on your health and well-being, so it is important to stay informed about potential complications and follow-up care. Your healthcare provider can help you understand what to expect in the months and years following surgery, as well as any steps you can take to minimize the risk of complications or recurrence. By staying proactive and engaged in your care, you can better manage the long-term effects of treatment and optimize your quality of life.

Finally, survivorship care planning may also involve connecting with support resources and organizations that can provide guidance, education, and emotional support. There are many resources available for patients with pituitary tumors, including support groups, online forums, and advocacy organizations that can help you navigate the challenges of living with a pituitary tumor. By staying informed and connected with others who understand your experience, you can better cope with the impact of pituitary tumors on your mental health and well-being.

Chapter 10: Support Resources for Patients with Pituitary Tumors

Patient Advocacy Organizations

Patient advocacy organizations play a crucial role in supporting individuals diagnosed with pituitary tumors. These organizations are dedicated to providing education, resources, and support to patients navigating the complexities of diagnosis and treatment. By connecting with patient advocacy organizations, individuals can access valuable information about their condition, treatment options, and ways to manage symptoms effectively. These organizations serve as a valuable ally for patients seeking guidance and assistance throughout their journey with pituitary tumors.

One of the key benefits of patient advocacy organizations is the wealth of information they provide about treatment options for pituitary tumors. Patients can learn about the various surgical interventions available, as well as non-invasive treatment methods that may be suitable for their specific case. By empowering patients with knowledge about their treatment options, advocacy organizations help individuals make informed decisions about their healthcare and advocate for the best possible outcomes.

In addition to treatment information, patient advocacy organizations also offer support resources for managing symptoms of pituitary tumors. From hormonal imbalances caused by the tumor to long-term effects of surgery, these organizations provide practical tips and strategies for coping with the physical and emotional challenges of living with a pituitary tumor. By connecting with others who understand their experience, patients can find comfort, reassurance, and a sense of community during difficult times.

Furthermore, patient advocacy organizations play a vital role in raising awareness about genetic factors related to pituitary tumors. By educating patients about the hereditary nature of these tumors, advocacy organizations help individuals make informed decisions about genetic testing and screening for themselves and their families. This information can be invaluable in understanding the risk of developing a pituitary tumor and taking proactive steps to prevent or detect the condition early.

Overall, patient advocacy organizations are a valuable resource for individuals living with pituitary tumors. From providing information on treatment options and managing symptoms to raising awareness about genetic factors and offering support resources, these organizations play a critical role in helping patients navigate the challenges of diagnosis and treatment. By connecting with advocacy organizations, patients can access the education, resources, and support they need to advocate for their health and well-being throughout their journey with a pituitary tumor.

Support Groups and Peer Networks

Support groups and peer networks can be invaluable resources for patients navigating the challenges of pituitary tumors. These groups provide a sense of community and understanding that can help patients feel less alone in their journey. By connecting with others who are facing similar struggles, patients can gain valuable insights, advice, and emotional support.

One of the benefits of participating in a support group is the opportunity to share experiences and learn from others who have gone through similar diagnoses and treatments. Hearing about others' successes and challenges can provide reassurance and help patients feel more empowered in managing their own healthcare. Support groups can also offer practical tips for coping with symptoms, navigating treatment options, and advocating for oneself within the healthcare system.

In addition to the emotional support and camaraderie that support groups provide, they can also be a valuable source of information. Members may share resources, research articles, and updates on new treatment options, helping patients stay informed and empowered in their healthcare decisions. Peer networks can also provide a platform for discussing topics such as hormonal imbalances, genetic factors, and long-term effects of pituitary tumor surgery, allowing patients to access a wealth of knowledge and expertise.

Support groups and peer networks can also play a crucial role in mental health and well-being for patients with pituitary tumors. Dealing with a chronic illness like a pituitary tumor can be overwhelming and isolating, leading to feelings of anxiety, depression, and stress. By connecting with others who understand their struggles, patients can find comfort, validation, and encouragement in their journey towards healing.

Overall, support groups and peer networks offer patients with pituitary tumors a safe space to share their experiences, gain knowledge, receive emotional support, and build a sense of community. Whether in-person or online, these resources can be instrumental in helping patients navigate the complexities of their diagnosis and treatment, and improve their overall quality of life.

Online Communities and Forums

Online communities and forums can be invaluable resources for patients navigating the complex world of pituitary tumors. These platforms provide a space for individuals to connect with others who are facing similar challenges, share experiences, and offer support and guidance. By joining an online community or forum dedicated to pituitary tumors, patients can gain valuable insights into their condition and learn about the latest treatment options and research developments.

One of the key benefits of participating in online communities and forums is the opportunity to learn about the various treatment options available for pituitary tumors. From surgical interventions to non-invasive treatment methods, patients can gain a better understanding of the pros and cons of each approach and make more informed decisions about their care. Additionally, these platforms can provide valuable information on managing symptoms and hormonal imbalances caused by pituitary tumors, helping patients improve their quality of life.

For patients considering surgical intervention for their pituitary tumor, online communities and forums can be a valuable source of support and information. Members of these communities can share their own experiences with surgery, offer tips for preparing for the procedure, and provide insights into the long-term effects of pituitary tumor surgery. By connecting with others who have been through similar experiences, patients can feel less alone and more empowered as they navigate their treatment journey.

In addition to practical information and support, online communities and forums can also provide a sense of community and belonging for patients with pituitary tumors. These platforms offer a safe space for individuals to share their fears, frustrations, and triumphs, and to connect with others who truly understand what they are going through. This sense of camaraderie can be incredibly comforting and empowering for patients, helping them feel less isolated and more supported in their journey.

Overall, online communities and forums can play a crucial role in helping patients with pituitary tumors navigate their diagnosis, treatment, and recovery. By connecting with others who share their experiences and insights, patients can gain valuable information, support, and encouragement as they face the challenges of living with a pituitary tumor. Whether seeking advice on treatment options, managing symptoms, or simply finding a sense of community, online platforms can be a valuable resource for patients looking to take control of their health and well-being.

Counseling and Therapy Services

Counseling and therapy services play a crucial role in the comprehensive care of patients with pituitary tumors. Navigating the diagnosis and treatment of pituitary tumors can be overwhelming and emotionally challenging for patients. Counseling and therapy services provide a safe space for patients to process their thoughts and emotions, cope with anxiety and stress, and develop effective coping strategies. These services are essential for promoting mental health and well-being throughout the journey of managing pituitary tumors.

Patients with pituitary tumors may experience a range of emotions, including fear, uncertainty, and grief. Counseling and therapy services can help patients navigate these complex emotions and develop resilience in the face of adversity. Therapists and counselors can provide emotional support, guidance, and practical tools to help patients cope with the challenges of living with a pituitary tumor. By addressing the psychological and emotional aspects of the disease, counseling and therapy services contribute to a holistic approach to patient care.

In addition to providing emotional support, counseling and therapy services can also help patients manage the symptoms of pituitary tumors. Patients may experience physical symptoms such as headaches, vision changes, fatigue, and hormonal imbalances, which can impact their quality of life. Therapists and counselors can work with patients to develop strategies for managing these symptoms, improving their overall well-being and quality of life.

Surgical interventions for pituitary tumors can have long-term effects on patients, both physically and emotionally. Counseling and therapy services can help patients navigate the emotional challenges of surgery, such as fear, anxiety, and adjustment to physical changes. Therapists and counselors can also support patients in coping with any long-term effects of surgery, such as hormonal imbalances or changes in body image. By providing ongoing emotional support and guidance, counseling and therapy services contribute to the overall well-being of patients post-surgery.

In conclusion, counseling and therapy services are an essential component of comprehensive care for patients with pituitary tumors. These services help patients navigate the emotional challenges of diagnosis and treatment, manage symptoms, cope with the effects of surgery, and improve their overall well-being. By addressing the psychological and emotional aspects of the disease, counseling and therapy services play a vital role in supporting patients throughout their journey of managing pituitary tumors.

Caregiver Support and Resources

Caregivers play a crucial role in supporting patients with pituitary tumors throughout their diagnosis and treatment journey. It is essential for caregivers to understand the complexities of pituitary tumors, the various treatment options available, and how to effectively manage the symptoms that may arise. By providing emotional support, assisting with daily tasks, and advocating for the patient's needs, caregivers can positively impact the patient's overall well-being.

One important aspect of caregiver support is being knowledgeable about the different treatment options for pituitary tumors. From surgical interventions to non-invasive treatment methods, caregivers should be aware of the potential benefits and risks associated with each option. This knowledge can help caregivers make informed decisions alongside the patient and healthcare team, ensuring the best possible outcome for the patient.

In addition to treatment options, caregivers should also be prepared to assist with managing the symptoms of pituitary tumors. From hormonal imbalances to long-term effects of surgery, caregivers play a vital role in helping patients cope with the physical and emotional challenges that may arise. By providing comfort, reassurance, and practical assistance, caregivers can help alleviate some of the burdens faced by patients with pituitary tumors.

Support resources for patients with pituitary tumors are also available to caregivers. These resources can provide valuable information, emotional support, and practical assistance to help caregivers navigate the complexities of caring for a loved one with a pituitary tumor. From support groups to online forums, caregivers can connect with others who understand their unique challenges and find the support they need to effectively care for the patient.

Ultimately, caregiver support and resources are essential components of the comprehensive care plan for patients with pituitary tumors. By being informed, proactive, and compassionate, caregivers can make a significant difference in the patient's journey towards healing and recovery. It is important for caregivers to prioritize self-care and seek out support for themselves as well, recognizing the impact that caring for a loved one with a pituitary tumor can have on their own mental health and well-being.

Chapter 11: Pituitary Tumor Recurrence and Prevention Strategies

Monitoring and Surveillance

Monitoring and surveillance are crucial aspects of managing pituitary tumors effectively. Regular monitoring allows healthcare providers to track the growth and progression of the tumor, as well as evaluate the effectiveness of treatment interventions. Surveillance involves a combination of imaging studies, hormonal testing, and clinical assessments to ensure that any changes in the tumor are detected early and appropriate actions are taken promptly.

Imaging studies such as MRI or CT scans are commonly used to monitor the size and location of pituitary tumors. These scans provide detailed images of the pituitary gland and surrounding structures, allowing healthcare providers to assess the tumor's response to treatment and detect any signs of progression. Regular imaging studies are typically scheduled every 6-12 months, depending on the individual's specific circumstances.

Hormonal testing is another essential component of monitoring pituitary tumors. Pituitary tumors can disrupt the normal production of hormones in the body, leading to hormonal imbalances that can cause a variety of symptoms. Regular blood tests are used to measure hormone levels and evaluate the effectiveness of hormone replacement therapy or other treatment interventions. Monitoring hormone levels allows healthcare providers to adjust treatment plans as needed to optimize the patient's hormonal balance.

In addition to imaging studies and hormonal testing, clinical assessments play a crucial role in monitoring pituitary tumors. Healthcare providers will regularly evaluate the patient's symptoms, overall health, and quality of life to assess the impact of the tumor and treatment interventions. These assessments help healthcare providers understand the patient's individual needs and make informed decisions about ongoing care and management.

Overall, monitoring and surveillance are essential components of managing pituitary tumors effectively. By staying vigilant and proactive in tracking the tumor's growth and progression, healthcare providers can optimize treatment outcomes and improve the patient's quality of life. Regular imaging studies, hormonal testing, and clinical assessments are key tools in this process, allowing healthcare providers to tailor treatment plans to meet the individual needs of each patient.

Recurrence Risk Factors

Understanding the risk factors for pituitary tumor recurrence is crucial for patients who have undergone treatment. While recurrence rates vary depending on the type and size of the tumor, as well as the treatment received, there are certain factors that can increase the likelihood of the tumor returning. By being aware of these risk factors, patients can work closely with their healthcare team to develop a proactive plan for monitoring and managing their condition.

One of the primary risk factors for pituitary tumor recurrence is the type of tumor itself. Certain types of pituitary tumors, such as invasive or aggressive tumors, are more likely to come back even after treatment. Additionally, the size of the tumor at the time of diagnosis can also play a role in recurrence risk. Larger tumors may be more difficult to completely remove during surgery, increasing the chances of residual tumor cells remaining.

Another important factor to consider is the level of hormonal activity associated with the tumor. Tumors that produce excess hormones, such as prolactin or growth hormone, may be more likely to recur if not effectively managed. Patients with functional tumors should work closely with an endocrinologist to monitor hormone levels and adjust medication as needed to reduce the risk of recurrence.

In some cases, genetic factors can also contribute to the risk of pituitary tumor recurrence. Patients with a family history of pituitary tumors or certain genetic syndromes may have a higher likelihood of developing tumors that are prone to recurrence. Genetic testing and counseling may be recommended for patients with a family history of pituitary tumors to better understand their individual risk factors.

Overall, a multidisciplinary approach to care is essential for managing the risk of pituitary tumor recurrence. Patients should stay vigilant in attending follow-up appointments with their healthcare team, including endocrinologists, neurosurgeons, and oncologists, to monitor for any signs of tumor regrowth. By working collaboratively with their providers and staying informed about their individual risk factors, patients can take proactive steps to minimize the chances of tumor recurrence and maintain their overall health and well-being.

Salvage Treatment Options

Salvage treatment options refer to additional treatment options that may be considered when initial treatments for pituitary tumors have not been successful or when the tumor has recurred. These options are typically used as a last resort to help manage symptoms and improve quality of life for patients. It is important for patients to work closely with their healthcare team to determine the best course of action for their specific situation.

One salvage treatment option for pituitary tumors is radiation therapy. Radiation therapy uses high-energy beams to target and destroy tumor cells. This treatment may be recommended if surgery and medication have not been effective in controlling tumor growth or if the tumor has come back after initial treatment. Radiation therapy can help shrink the tumor and reduce symptoms, but it may also have side effects that patients should discuss with their healthcare team.

Another salvage treatment option for pituitary tumors is chemotherapy. Chemotherapy uses drugs to kill cancer cells and may be used in cases where other treatments have not been successful. Chemotherapy is typically not a first-line treatment for pituitary tumors, but it may be considered in certain situations. Patients should be aware of the potential side effects of chemotherapy and work closely with their healthcare team to monitor their response to treatment.

In some cases, hormonal therapy may be used as a salvage treatment option for pituitary tumors. Hormonal therapy involves taking medications to help regulate hormone levels in the body and may be used to manage symptoms caused by hormonal imbalances. This treatment may be used in conjunction with other treatments to help control tumor growth and improve quality of life for patients.

It is important for patients with pituitary tumors to discuss salvage treatment options with their healthcare team and make informed decisions about their care. Patients should be proactive in seeking out information and support resources to help them navigate their diagnosis and treatment. By working closely with their healthcare team and staying informed about their options, patients can better manage their symptoms and improve their overall well-being.

Lifestyle Modifications

Lifestyle modifications play a crucial role in managing pituitary tumors and improving overall health for patients. Making small changes in daily habits can have a significant impact on the progression of the tumor and the management of symptoms. By adopting a healthy lifestyle, patients can support their treatment plan and enhance their quality of life.

Diet and nutrition are key components of lifestyle modifications for patients with pituitary tumors. A well-balanced diet rich in fruits, vegetables, whole grains, and lean proteins can help support the body's immune system and promote healing. Patients should also aim to reduce their intake of processed foods, sugary drinks, and high-fat foods, as these can contribute to inflammation and other health issues. Staying hydrated and limiting caffeine intake can also help manage symptoms such as headaches and fatigue.

Regular exercise is another important lifestyle modification for patients with pituitary tumors. Physical activity can help improve mood, reduce stress, and increase energy levels. Patients should work with their healthcare team to develop an exercise plan that is safe and appropriate for their individual needs. Incorporating activities such as walking, swimming, or yoga can help improve overall strength and flexibility.

Managing stress is essential for patients with pituitary tumors, as stress can exacerbate symptoms and impact overall well-being. Practicing relaxation techniques such as deep breathing, meditation, or mindfulness can help reduce stress levels and improve mental health. Patients may also benefit from seeking support from a therapist or counselor to address any emotional challenges they may face.

In addition to diet, exercise, and stress management, patients with pituitary tumors should prioritize adequate sleep and rest. Getting enough sleep is crucial for healing and maintaining overall health. Patients should establish a regular sleep routine, create a comfortable sleep environment, and practice good sleep hygiene habits. By implementing these lifestyle modifications, patients can support their treatment plan, manage symptoms, and improve their quality of life while navigating the challenges of living with a pituitary tumor.

Survivorship Care Planning

Survivorship care planning is an essential aspect of managing pituitary tumors, as it involves developing a comprehensive plan to address the physical, emotional, and psychological needs of patients after treatment. This plan aims to help patients navigate the post-treatment phase, manage potential side effects, and maintain their overall well-being. By addressing these aspects of survivorship care, patients can improve their quality of life and reduce the risk of tumor recurrence.

One of the key components of survivorship care planning is understanding the long-term effects of pituitary tumor surgery. Surgery is often a necessary treatment option for pituitary tumors, but it can lead to hormonal imbalances and other complications that require ongoing management. Patients should work closely with their healthcare team to monitor these effects and develop a plan for addressing any issues that may arise in the future.

In addition to surgical interventions, there are non-invasive treatment methods available for managing pituitary tumors. These treatments, such as radiation therapy or medication, can help control tumor growth and alleviate symptoms without the need for surgery. Patients should discuss these options with their healthcare team to determine the most appropriate course of treatment for their individual needs.

Managing the symptoms of pituitary tumors is another important aspect of survivorship care planning. These symptoms can vary depending on the type and location of the tumor, but may include headaches, vision changes, fatigue, and hormonal imbalances. Patients should work with their healthcare team to develop strategies for managing these symptoms and improving their overall quality of life.

In conclusion, survivorship care planning plays a crucial role in helping patients navigate the challenges of living with a pituitary tumor. By addressing the long-term effects of treatment, exploring non-invasive treatment options, and managing symptoms effectively, patients can improve their overall well-being and reduce the risk of tumor recurrence. It is important for patients to be proactive in their care and work closely with their healthcare team to develop a personalized survivorship care plan that meets their individual needs.

Chapter 12: Impact of Pituitary Tumors on Mental Health and Well-Being

Depression and Anxiety

Depression and anxiety are common mental health challenges faced by patients with pituitary tumors. The impact of these tumors on hormone production can lead to hormonal imbalances that contribute to mood disorders. It is important for patients to recognize the signs and symptoms of depression and anxiety, as well as seek support from healthcare providers and mental health professionals.

Patients with pituitary tumors may experience feelings of sadness, hopelessness, and anxiety due to the physical and emotional challenges associated with their condition. These symptoms can be exacerbated by the stress of navigating diagnosis and treatment options. It is crucial for patients to communicate openly with their healthcare team about their mental health concerns, as addressing these issues can improve overall quality of life and treatment outcomes.

Treatment options for pituitary tumors may include surgical interventions, non-invasive treatment methods, and hormonal therapies. These treatments can have a significant impact on a patient's physical and emotional well-being. It is common for patients to experience anxiety and depression before and after surgery, as well as during recovery. Healthcare providers should be proactive in assessing and addressing the mental health needs of patients throughout their treatment journey.

Managing symptoms of pituitary tumors, such as fatigue, cognitive difficulties, and changes in mood, can be challenging for patients. It is important for patients to prioritize self-care and seek support from loved ones and healthcare providers. Engaging in activities that promote relaxation and stress reduction, such as mindfulness meditation and gentle exercise, can help alleviate symptoms of depression and anxiety.

Support resources for patients with pituitary tumors, such as online forums, support groups, and counseling services, can provide valuable emotional support and coping strategies. Patients are encouraged to connect with others who are facing similar challenges and share their experiences. By taking an active role in their mental health and well-being, patients can better navigate the emotional impact of pituitary tumors and improve their overall quality of life.

Body Image and Self-Esteem

Body image and self-esteem can be greatly affected by a pituitary tumor diagnosis and treatment. Patients may experience physical changes due to hormonal imbalances caused by the tumor, such as weight gain, hair loss, or changes in skin condition. These changes can impact how patients see themselves and may lead to a decrease in self-esteem. It is important to remember that these changes are a result of the tumor and its treatment, and do not define your worth as a person.

Managing symptoms of pituitary tumors can also play a role in body image and self-esteem. Some symptoms, such as fatigue, mood swings, or headaches, can impact how patients feel about themselves and their ability to function on a daily basis. It is important to communicate with your healthcare team about any symptoms you are experiencing so they can help you manage them effectively. This can help improve your overall quality of life and boost your self-esteem.

Surgical interventions for pituitary tumors may also impact body image and self-esteem. Depending on the location and size of the tumor, surgery may result in visible scars or changes in facial appearance. It is important to discuss these potential changes with your healthcare team before undergoing surgery so you can prepare mentally and emotionally. Remember that these changes are a small price to pay for potentially life-saving treatment.

Non-invasive treatment methods for pituitary tumors, such as medication or radiation therapy, may also have an impact on body image and self-esteem. Some medications may cause weight gain or changes in skin condition, while radiation therapy may lead to fatigue or hair loss. It is important to discuss any concerns you have about these treatments with your healthcare team so they can provide support and guidance.

Overall, it is important to remember that your body image and self-esteem are not solely determined by physical appearance. Your worth as a person is not defined by the changes caused by a pituitary tumor or its treatment. It is important to focus on self-care, self-acceptance, and seeking support from your healthcare team and loved ones. Remember that you are not alone in this journey, and there are resources available to help you navigate the challenges of a pituitary tumor diagnosis and treatment.

Coping Strategies and Resilience

When faced with a diagnosis of a pituitary tumor, it is normal to experience a range of emotions, including fear, anxiety, and uncertainty. Coping with the physical and emotional challenges of living with a pituitary tumor can be overwhelming, but developing effective coping strategies and resilience is essential for navigating this journey.

One important coping strategy is to educate yourself about pituitary tumors and their treatment options. By understanding your condition and the various treatment approaches available, you can make informed decisions about your care and feel more empowered in managing your health. This knowledge can also help alleviate some of the anxiety and uncertainty that often accompany a pituitary tumor diagnosis.

In addition to educating yourself, it is important to seek support from healthcare providers, family, friends, and support groups. Connecting with others who have experienced similar challenges can provide valuable insights, encouragement, and a sense of community. Building a strong support network can also help you feel less isolated and more hopeful as you navigate the complexities of living with a pituitary tumor.

Practicing self-care is another crucial coping strategy for managing the symptoms and side effects of a pituitary tumor. Prioritizing healthy habits such as regular exercise, nutritious eating, adequate sleep, and stress management can help improve your overall well-being and resilience. Engaging in activities that bring you joy and relaxation, such as hobbies, meditation, or spending time in nature, can also help reduce stress and enhance your coping abilities.

Developing resilience in the face of a pituitary tumor diagnosis involves cultivating a positive mindset and adaptive coping skills. This may include practicing mindfulness, gratitude, and acceptance of your circumstances, as well as maintaining a sense of humor and optimism. Building resilience is an ongoing process that requires patience, perseverance, and self-compassion, but it can help you navigate the challenges of living with a pituitary tumor with greater strength and adaptability.

In conclusion, coping strategies and resilience are essential for managing the physical, emotional, and psychological aspects of living with a pituitary tumor. By educating yourself, seeking support, practicing self-care, and developing resilience, you can enhance your ability to cope with the challenges of your condition and navigate your treatment journey with greater confidence and well-being. Remember that you are not alone in this journey, and there are resources and support available to help you every step of the way.

Social Relationships and Support Systems

Social relationships and support systems play a crucial role in navigating the complexities of pituitary tumors. As a patient facing this diagnosis, it is important to recognize the impact that your relationships with family, friends, and healthcare providers can have on your journey towards healing. These individuals can provide emotional support, practical assistance, and valuable information to help you make informed decisions about your treatment options.

When facing a pituitary tumor diagnosis, it is common to experience a range of emotions, including fear, anxiety, and uncertainty. Having a strong support system in place can help alleviate some of these feelings and provide a sense of comfort during this challenging time. Whether it is through listening ear, helping hand, or simply being present, the people in your life can offer a sense of stability and reassurance as you navigate the ups and downs of treatment.

In addition to the emotional support provided by loved ones, it is also important to seek out support resources specifically tailored to patients with pituitary tumors. These resources can include support groups, online forums, and educational materials that can help you connect with others who are going through similar experiences. By sharing your journey with others who understand what you are going through, you can gain valuable insights, advice, and encouragement to help you cope with the challenges of living with a pituitary tumor.

Furthermore, support systems can also play a role in helping you manage the physical symptoms of pituitary tumors. Whether it is assisting with transportation to medical appointments, helping with household tasks, or providing a listening ear when you are feeling unwell, having a strong support network can make it easier to cope with the day-to-day challenges of living with a pituitary tumor. By enlisting the help of others, you can focus on your healing and well-being, knowing that you are not alone in your journey.

Overall, social relationships and support systems are essential components of a comprehensive treatment plan for pituitary tumors. By nurturing these connections and seeking out support resources, you can empower yourself to make informed decisions about your care, manage your symptoms effectively, and improve your overall quality of life. Remember, you do not have to face this diagnosis alone – reach out to those around you for help, guidance, and encouragement as you navigate the complexities of living with a pituitary tumor.

Integrative Therapies and Holistic Approaches

Integrative Therapies and Holistic Approaches play a crucial role in the overall management of pituitary tumors. These complementary treatment options can help patients navigate their diagnosis and treatment journey more effectively, while also addressing the physical, emotional, and mental aspects of living with a pituitary tumor. Integrative therapies focus on treating the whole person, rather than just the disease, and can provide valuable support alongside traditional medical interventions.

One of the key benefits of incorporating integrative therapies into your treatment plan is the potential to manage symptoms of pituitary tumors more effectively. Therapies such as acupuncture, massage therapy, and meditation have been shown to help alleviate pain, reduce stress and anxiety, and improve overall quality of life for patients with pituitary tumors. These holistic approaches can complement medical treatments and help patients cope with the physical and emotional challenges of living with a pituitary tumor.

In addition to symptom management, integrative therapies can also help address hormonal imbalances caused by pituitary tumors. Certain therapies, such as dietary modifications, herbal supplements, and mind-body practices, can support hormone regulation and improve overall endocrine function. By working in tandem with traditional medical treatments, integrative therapies can help optimize hormone levels and enhance the effectiveness of treatment for pituitary tumors.

Furthermore, integrative therapies can play a role in preventing pituitary tumor recurrence. By focusing on overall health and wellness, these holistic approaches can support the body's natural healing processes and reduce the likelihood of tumor regrowth. Patients who incorporate integrative therapies into their long-term care plan may experience improved outcomes and reduced risk of tumor recurrence, leading to better overall prognosis and quality of life.

Overall, integrating holistic approaches into your treatment plan can have a positive impact on your mental health and well-being as you navigate the challenges of living with a pituitary tumor. These therapies can help promote relaxation, reduce anxiety, and improve coping mechanisms, ultimately enhancing your overall quality of life. By exploring integrative therapies alongside traditional medical treatments, patients with pituitary tumors can take a comprehensive and personalized approach to their care, addressing their unique needs and supporting their journey towards health and healing.

Conclusion: Empowering Patients to Navigate Diagnosis and Treatment of Pituitary Tumors

In conclusion, empowering patients to navigate the diagnosis and treatment of pituitary tumors is crucial in ensuring the best possible outcomes for individuals facing this challenging condition. By arming themselves with knowledge and understanding of their condition, patients can actively participate in their care and make informed decisions about their treatment options.

Patients facing pituitary tumors must be aware of the various treatment options available to them, ranging from surgical interventions to non-invasive methods. By working closely with their healthcare team, patients can determine the most appropriate course of action based on their unique circumstances and preferences.

Managing the symptoms of pituitary tumors is another important aspect of patient empowerment. By understanding the potential hormonal imbalances caused by these tumors and working with their medical team to address these issues, patients can improve their quality of life and overall well-being.

Furthermore, patients should be aware of the long-term effects of pituitary tumor surgery and take steps to minimize potential complications. By staying informed and proactive in their follow-up care, patients can reduce the risk of recurrence and ensure optimal recovery.

Finally, patients should take advantage of support resources available to them, whether it be through support groups, counseling services, or online communities. By seeking out these resources and building a strong support network, patients can better cope with the emotional and psychological impact of pituitary tumors and maintain their mental health and well-being throughout their journey.